Oral Controlled
Release Products
Gundert-Remy/Möller

Paperback APV

Die Buchreihe wird im Auftrag der Arbeitsgemeinschaft für Pharmazeutische Verfahrenstechnik e.V. (APV), Mainz, herausgegeben.

Band 22

In der Reihe Paperback APV sind bereits erschienen:

Band 1 Hauschild
Ausgangsmaterialien für die Arzneimittelherstellung. Qualitätsforderungen (GMP) und deren Folgen für Zulieferer und Pharma-Betriebe

Band 2 Essig/Schmidt/Stumpf
Flüssige Arzneimittelformen und Arzneimittelsicherheit. Unter besonderer Berücksichtigung der Qualität von Wasser

Band 3 Hasler
Dosierungsgenauigkeit einzeldosierter fester Arzneiformen

Band 4 Brandau/Lippold
Dermal and Transdermal Absorption

Band 5 Schrank/Skinner
Arzneimittelhygiene von der Herstellung bis zur Verabreichung

Band 6 Oeser
Selbstinspektion und Inspektion. GMP-Forderungen zur Qualitätssicherung im Arzneimittel-Bereich

Band 7 Fahrig/Hofer
Die Kapsel. Grundlagen, Technologie und Biopharmazie einer modernen Arzneiform

Band 8 Sucker
Praxis der Validierung unter besonderer Berücksichtigung der FIP-Richtlinien für die gute Validierungspraxis

Band 9 Algner/Helbig/Spingler
Primär-Packmittel. Herstellung + Optimierung + Kontrolle = Sicherheit

Band 10 Asche/Essig/Schmidt
Technologie von Salben, Suspensionen und Emulsionen

Band 11 Hanke
Qualität pflanzlicher Arzneimittel. Prüfung und Herstellung – Anforderungen bei der Zulassung

Band 12 Dertinger/Gänshirt/Steinigen
GAP – Praxisgerechtes Arbeiten in pharmazeutisch-analysierten Laboratorien

Band 13 Helbig/Singler
Kunststoffe für die Pharmazeutische Verpackung. Einsatz – Anforderungen – Prüfverfahren

Band 14 Brandau
Pharmaproduktion aus betriebswirtschaftlicher Sicht

Band 15 Essig/Hofer/Schmidt/Stumpf
Stabilisierungstechnologie
Wege zur haltbaren Arzneiform

Band 16 Grimm
Stability Testing of Pharmaceutical Products

Band 17 Müller
Controlled Drug Delivery

Band 18 Schultz/Grünewald
Strahlen- und Gassterilisation

Band 19 Hauschild/Spingler
Migration bei Kunststoffverpackungen

Band 20 Altenschmidt/Hasler/Möller
Probenahme bei der Qualitätssicherung von Arzneimitteln

Oral Controlled Release Products

Therapeutic and Biopharmaceutic Assessment

Edited by
Prof. Dr. U. Gundert-Remy
Bundesgesundheitsamt, Berlin

and
Priv.-Doz. Dr. H. Möller
Hoechst AG, Frankfurt

with 83 figures and 9 tables

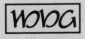

Wissenschaftliche Verlagsgesellschaft mbH Stuttgart 1990

Ein Markenzeichen kann warenzeichenrechtlich geschützt sein, auch wenn ein Hinweis auf etwa bestehende Schutzrechte fehlt.

Deutsche Bibliothek Cataloguing-in-Publication Data

Oral controlled release products: therapeutic and biopharmaceutic assessment / ed. by U. Gundert-Remy and H. Möller. – Stuttgart: Wiss. Verl.-Ges., 1989
  (Paperback APV; Bd. 22)
  ISBN 3-8047-1042-5
NE: Gundert-Remy, Ursula [Hrsg.]; Arbeitsgemeinschaft für Pharmazeutische Verfahrenstechnik: Paperback APV

© 1990 Wissenschaftliche Verlagsgesellschaft mbH, Birkenwaldstraße 44, 7000 Stuttgart 1
Printed in Germany
Satz und Druck: Röck, Weinsberg
Umschlaggestaltung: Hans Hug, Stuttgart

Contents

A. Preface   7

B. Contributors   9

C. Lectures   11

   I. Controlled Release Products – Therapeutic Aspects   13
      (U. Gundert-Remy, D-Berlin)

  II. Controlled Release Products – Pharmacokinetic Aspects   21
      (L. Balant, CH-Genf)

 III. Controlled Release Products – Approaches of Pharmaceutical
      Technology   39
      (B. Lippold, D-Düsseldorf)

  IV. Gastro-Intestinal Absorption and Transportkinetics   59
      (H. Möller, D-Frankfurt)

   V. Chronopharmacology as a Rationale for the Development of
      Controlled Release Products   83
      (H. Staudinger, D-Konstanz)

  VI. Pharmacokinetic Characteristics of Controlled Release
      Products and their Biostatistical Analysis   99
      (V. Steinijans, D-Konstanz)

 VII. The Significance of Nutrition for the Biopharmaceutical
      Characteristics of Oral Controlled Release Products and
      Enteric Coated Dosage Forms 117
      (I. Walter–Sack, D-Heidelberg)

VIII. In vitro-Dissolution Testing of Oral Controlled Release
      Products 139
      (M. Siewert, D-Eschborn)

  IX. Association Between in Vitro and in Vivo 155
      (M. Nicklasson, S-Solna)

X. Regulatory Recommendations in USA on Investigation and
Evaluation of Oral Controlled Release Products 175
(J. Skelly, USA-Rockville)
XI. Regulatory Recommendations in Europe on Investigation
and Evaluation of Oral Controlled Release Products. 195
(A. G. Rauws, M. Olling, NL-Bilthoven)

A
Preface

Over the past decades a huge number of oral, controlled release products have been marketed with the aim of prolonging the therapeutic effect by extending the release of the drug substance from different types of galenical dosage forms. Advantages of this kind of dosage form are to be seen in the reduced dosing frequency and in the improvement in patient compliance. Moreover, the plasma concentration-time profiles of these dosage forms tend to fluctuate less, thereby reducing side effects related to the high peak concentrations which result from the use of immediate release products.

Controlled release products are defined by the F.D.A. as those formulations designed to release an active constituent at rates which differ significantly from those of their corresponding immediate release forms. Many terms have been used to describe these forms; e. g. delayed release, extended release, gradual release, modified release, prolonged release, protracted release, repeat action, slow release, sustained release, depot, retard and time release dosage forms.

Any of these or similar terms which impart the same idea may be used to define the controlled release product. Generally, efforts should be made to use only one term; e. g. controlled release product, which conveys the galenical concept behind the controlled release form, i. e. avoidance of physiological interference in release behaviour caused by the pH and the motility of the gastro-intestinal tract.

For this reason, the term "controlled release product" is used throughout.

This book summarizes the lectures held at the APV symposium in June 1988, Würzburg, and covers the main aspects of pharmacodynamic, pharmacokinetic and physico-chemical characterisation of controlled release forms. The latter aspect may be seen in relation to the concept of pharmaceutical and technological design of controlled release patterns.

Suitable pharmacokinetic characteristics are needed to assess and compare in vivo the controlled release of different formulations. Apart from the known, conventional characteristics, additional characteristics are considered which meet the requirements laid down by the authorities responsible for approval procedures and which guarantee the comparable evaluation of marketed products. Therefore, reference is made to the regulatory recommendations of the USA and the EC. New guidelines are in preparation in the USA, the EC and Japan and we sincerely hope that they will become international standards. This book is intended to be of help in this process.

Several aspects should be taken into consideration during the development of controlled release products viz. time dependencies of absorption and transport kinetics of the dosage form, chronopharmacology, influence of nutrition and the association between in vivo and in vitro-dissolution. The in vitro-dissolution method, validated by means of in vivo data, guarantees that the marketed controlled release product meets the requirements of quality control.

Prof. Dr. U. Gundert-Remy and Priv.-Doz. Dr. H. Möller

B
Contributors

Dr. L. Balant
Universitätsklinik Genf
Abteilung für Psychiatrie
Postfach 79

CH-1211 Genf 8

Prof. Dr. U. Gundert-Remy
Bundesgesundheitsamt
Institut für Arzneimittel
Seestraße 10

D-1000 Berlin 65

Prof. Dr. B. C. Lippold
Institut für Pharmazeutische
Technologie der Universität Düsseldorf
Universitätsstraße 1
Gebäude 26.22

D-4000 Düsseldorf 1

Priv.-Doz. Dr. H. Möller
Hoechst AG
Postfach 800320
Brüningstraße 50

D-6230 Frankfurt/Main 80

Prof. Dr. M. Nicklasson
Kabi Pharma
P. O. Box 1828

S-171 26 Solna

Dr. A. G. Rauws
National Institute of Public Health
and Environmental Protection
P. O. Box 1
Antonie van Leeuwenhoeklaan 9

NL-3720 BA Bilthoven

Dr. Siewert
Zentrallaboratorium Deutscher
Apotheker
Ginnheimer Straße 20

D-6236 Eschborn/Ts.

Dr. J. Skelly
Food and Drug Administration
Division of Biopharmaceutics
Center for Drugs and Biologics
5600 Fishers Lane Rm. 16–72

USA-Rockville MD 20857

Dr. H. Staudinger
Byk Gulden Lomberg
Chemische Fabrik GmbH
Postfach 6500
Byk-Gulden-Straße 2

D-7500 Konstanz

Dr. V. Steinijans
Byk Gulden Lomberg
Chemische Fabrik GmbH
Postfach 6500
Byk-Gulden-Straße 2

D-7750 Konstanz

Priv.-Doz. Dr. I. Walter-Sack
Medizinische Universitätsklinik
Abteilung für Klinische Pharmakologie
Bergheimer Straße 58

D-6900 Heidelberg 1

C
Lectures

I. Controlled Release Products – Therapeutic Aspects

Ursula Gundert-Remy, Berlin

Summary

From the therapeutic point of view the following reasons can be given to justify the development of a controlled release form: 1. better compliance, 2. prevention of unwanted effects, 3. maintenance of a therapeutic effect over an extended dosage interval without producing large fluctuations.

Contrasted with these advantages are the following possible disadvantages: 1. reduction in the amount absorbed/systemically available, 2. dose dumping, 3. higher variability of the amount absorbed/systemically available, 4. possible development of tolerance.

In this review the positive and negative aspects are examined by screening reports from the literature. It can be concluded that the possible advantages of a controlled release form should be proven in each individual case because they are not necessarily obtained from the available data in a manner in which they can be extrapolated without experimental proof. The disadvantages are well founded in theory and are demonstrated by various reports. However, it is justified to assume that they can be overcome partly by the use of suitable pharmaceutical technology. The problem of the development of tolerance should be interpreted as a problem of the dosage interval rather than a problem of controlled release forms.

1. General considerations

When developing a new chemical compound, the route leads from the synthesis of a new molecule first to studies in in-vitro models and experimental animal models assuming that these models will reveal effects which could be of therapeutic benefit. The synthesis of the new molecule is often guided by previous knowledge of similar molecules whose effects and in some cases therapeutic efficacy are known.

When developing the substance further, a decision has to be made as to whether to use it in humans after having carried out toxicological studies in animals. If the initial trials in humans give favourable results, therapeutic testing in the form of use in patients with a certain target disease enables the therapeutic suitability of the molecule to be assessed. When evaluating the therapeutic suitability, favourable effects on the course of the disease must be weighed up against the undesirable effects which occur after administration of the drug.

A study of the pharmacological textbooks, reference works and standard literature on a certain drug generally reveals information on the **active drug substance** but does not give details of the **pharmaceutical preparation,** after which the reported effects and side effects occurred.

In these references, the question as to whether a certain **dosage form** determines the duration and intensity of the effects observed, irrespective of whether they are assessed as desirable effects within the context of therapeutic use, is rarely posed or even mentioned.

Thus the dosage form, particularly a special galenical formulation with delayed release of the active substance, is not the primary aim of developing a new molecule into a drug, nor is it the focus of scientific discussions on a new chemical entity. Nevertheless, if the new drug compound has been marketed, the aspect of developing a controlled release form might arise and the pro's and con's have to be discussed.

Using the available literature as a basis, the aim of this report is to investigate aspects from which the development of a controlled release formulation can be regarded as a therapeutically sound means of improving treatment. Similarly, aspects are discussed which can be put forward as therapeutic disadvantages militating against the development of a controlled release formulation.

2. Points in favour of the use of controlled release products

2.1 Patient compliance

From the mid-70s onwards the problem of patient compliance has been discussed in German-speaking countries as an important variable in drug therapy. Reducing the times when the drug has to be taken and thereby improving compliance was and still is an argument in favour of the development of dosage forms with delayed release of the active substance. Nevertheless, a search through the literature reveals only a very few studies in which the authors not only claim to have improved compliance but have also attempted to demonstrate it experimentally. Thus a report by Tabachnik et al. (24)

(1982) showed that compliance in children was slightly better with a controlled-release formulation of theophylline than with a conventional dosage form. On the other hand a study by Taylor et al. (25) (1984) in adults indicates that the compliance of patients, most of whom received theophylline in controlled release form, was not better than is described in the literature. In a well-designed study Baird et al. (2) demonstrated that the compliance rate in patients who received controlled release metoprolol once a day was better than that in patients who had to take a conventional form twice daily. As regards the therapeutic efficacy there was no difference in the systolic and diastolic blood pressure, which is due to the fact that the difference in the compliance rates was statistically significant but only slightly pronounced.

2.2 Prevention of unwanted drug side effects

The precondition for the development of a controlled release form with the aim to prevent unwanted side effects is the establishment of a concentration/effect relationship to show that exceeding a specific concentration for a short time is associated with unwanted effects. Another possible background that is theoretically conceivable would be the connection between the triggering of undesirable effects and the rate of increase in the plasma concentration.

An association between the steepness of the increase in the plasma level and the triggering of unwanted effects in the form of tachycardia was demonstrated for nifedipine by the group of Breimer (14, 15).

Gastrointestinal side effects after nifedipine were however just as common in a study with healthy subjects who received tablets in a controlled release form as after rapid-release capsules and did not appear to correlate with the plasma level. However drowsiness was reported less often in this study (21) when nifedipine had been given in controlled release form.

In a review of controlled release dosage forms of beta-blockers (11) the authors explain that in comparative studies the incidence of undesirable side effects with controlled release forms is usually lower than with conventional forms and associate this with a lower peak concentration, without quoting a reference. However the only report which could be found in a search of the literature (2) did not bear this out. Undesirable side effects were just as common with a controlled release form of metoprolol as they were with a conventional dosage form. Unwanted effects occured in 86 out of 193 patients with the controlled release formulation and in 71 out of 196 patients with the conventional formulation.

Just as speculative as the reduction in undesirable effects as a result of the administration of controlled release beta-blockers are the investigations into the lower incidence of unwanted effects after depot neuroleptic agents (7). With trihexyphenidyl on the other hand it was shown that the intensity and frequency of some unwanted effects were reduced after administration in controlled release form (5).

There are a number of controlled release forms of NSAIDS on the market. But no relationship between concentration and effect, including undesirable effects, has been established, except in the case of a few substances (8). With salicylates it was demonstrated that the blood loss in the faeces (9) and unwanted gastrointestinal effects (19) after the administration of enteric-coated forms were less frequent than after conventional ASA.

Indomethacin is another drug which has been thoroughly investigated in this respect. Reports by Baber et al. (1), Kaarela et al. (13) and Düsing et al. (4) suggest that the incidence of symptoms of the central nervous system is lower after the administration of indomethacin in controlled release form than after its administration in immediate release form. Nevertheless Green (27) is of the opinion that nothing is to be gained from the controlled release form in terms of the avoidance of unwanted effects because this could not be demonstrated in a number of other studies.

Lithium is another example of contradictory results. Here details of a lower incidence of unwanted effects (18) are contrasted with a report on the triggering of diarrhoea (6). A rational explanation cannot be given for the findings of Wilder et al. (26) who observed a lower incidence of undesirable effects after the administration of an enteric-coated form of valproate than after the administration of a conventional form. Apart from the fact that the time of the maximum plasma level was postponed by two hours because of a two-hour lag-time, no difference was determined between the two forms in terms of the maximum level, the steepness of the increase and the area under the courve.

2.3 Maintenance of a therapeutic level over a prolonged period of time with only slight fluctuations

The argument that the problem of extreme fluctuations in the plasma level can be overcome by means of a changed formulation is certainly true in theory. For some active substance therapeutic concentration ranges have been defined, within which the plasma levels were said to be favourable.

Evidence that a controlled release of the active substance has therapeutic advantages over a conventional rapid release form has been tested by measuring the levels. Theophylline is a widely used example as an active substance (12).

Another example of a possible favourable effect of a controlled release form ist the less pronounced maximum sodium excretion with the absence of a rebound phenomenon after the administration of frusemide in controlled release form to healthy subjects (16). This could be attributed to the fact that after the administration of frusemide in controlled release form a more uniform diuretic effect is achieved. A comparison of the volumes of urine suggests this but the assessment of the findings is complicated by the fact that, in the paper quoted, frusemide in conventional form ist compared with frusemide retard plus 50 mg triamterene.

Likewise, for propanolol, after administration of a single dose, a difference between the conventional and two controlled release formulations was determined in terms of the duration of effect, measured on the basis of the reduction in exercise induced tachycardia (20). But in the steady state the difference between the formulations was reduced to such an extent that this could no longer be interpreted as relevant from the medical point of view.

3. Possible disadvantages of drugs with controlled release of the active substance

3.1 Reduction in the amount absorbed/systemically available

As the effectiveness of the absorption in the lower intestinal tract decreases, a reduction in the amount of the dose that is available in the body is to be expected with a programmed release over the entire gastrointestinal tract. Examples of this are studies carried out with propanolol (17, 22) and theophylline (10)

3.2 Dumping problem

The single dose of a form with controlled release of the active substance usually contains a multiple of the single dose of a rapid release form; this applies particularly to drugs with a very short half-life. A sudden, unexpected immediate release of the active substance can give rise to symptoms of intoxication. This has been discussed particularly in connection with theophylline-containing drugs for once-daily administration.

3.3 Problem of variability

Because of the relatively complex processes which can play a role when the drug is to be absorbed over the whole length of the intestine, such as intestinal motility, pH conditions and other factors, higher variability is to be expected after the administration of controlled release preparations. This is true of some of the controlled release preparations but not all (12, 20). Whether the degrees of variability observed are of clinical significance still has to be established.

3.4 Possible development of tolerance

Development of tolerance of the unwanted effects of organic nitrates has been known for almost a hundred years, at least in terms of the fall in blood pressure and the triggering of headaches. Several study groups showed that tolerance also develops to the therapeutic anti-anginal benefit of these drugs, especially in the case of long-term use of controlled release nitrate preparations: Thus the drug become clinically ineffective. However this development of tolerance can be prevented by changing the frequency of application so that the administration of a single high dose or the administration twice within six hours can be considered as a possible therapeutic regimen (3).

4. Conclusions

If the arguments for and against the development of a controlled-release form are summarized, it can be said that both the arguments in favour and the arguments against are well-founded in theory. The possible advantages in terms of compliance have not so far been adequately demonstrated by experimental data so this argument cannot be based on analogy with existing data without considering each case on its own merits. The argument of reducing or avoiding unwanted side effects can only be decisive if the corresponding studies bear it out and it is not an argument that can be generally used. The advantages of longerlasting and less fluctuating levels are in my view also often overinterpreted in discussion – for the majority of drugs at least there are no reliable clinical studies which demonstrate this advantage on the basis of clinical parameters.

On the other hand it must be admitted that the theoretically conceivable disadvantages of a controlled release formulation are also insufficiently substantiated by experimental clinical data.

Moreover, the problems of reduced absorption, dose dumping and increased variability can be overcome by good galenical development. The problem of the possible development of tolerance is certainly not due solely to the delayed release of the active substance but is also a matter of suitable dosage intervals.

From the review of the literature it can be concluded that controlled release forms can have advantages which should be demonstrated in each individual case and that on the other hand they can also have disadvantages, the absence of which also needs to be demonstrated.

5. Literature

(1) Baber, N., Halliday, L. D. C., Van den Heuvel, W. J. A., Walker, R. W., Sibeon, R., Keenan, J. P., Littler, T., Orme. M.: Indomethacin in rheumatoid arthritis: clinical effects, pharmacokinetics and platelet studies in responders and nonresponders. Ann. Rheum. Dis. 38, 128–137 (1979)

(2) Baird, M. G., Bentley-Taylor, M. M., Carruthers, S. G., Dawson, K. G., Laplante, L. E., Larochelle, P., MacCanell, K. L., Marquez-Julio, A., Silverberg, L. R., Talbot, P.: A Study of efficacy, tolerance and compliance of once-daily versus twice-daily metoprolol (Betaloc^R) in hypertension. Clinical & Investigative Medicine 7, 95–102 (1984)

(3) Blasini, R., Reininger, G., Rudolph, W.: Vermeidung einer Toleranzentwicklung bei Langzeittherapie mit Nitraten durch korrekte Dosierung. Z. Kardiol. 75, Suppl. 3, 42–49 (1986)

(4) Düsing, R., Dittrich, P., Kukovetz, W. R., Lehmann, K., Kramer, H. J.: Indomethacin-Kinetik und Urinausscheidung von Prostaglandin E_2 nach oraler Gabe verschiedener Indomethacin-Darreichungsformen. Z. Rheumatol. 42, 235–241 (1983)

(5) Devissaguet, J. P., Garbarg, S., Prost, M., Bogaievsky, Y.: Etude pharmacocinétique comparative de deux formes galéniques de trihexyphenidyle dosees à 5 mg comprimés (Artane^R) et gélules à liberation progressive (Parkinane retard^R). Thérapie 39, 231–236 (1984)

(6) Ehrlich, B. E., Diamond, J. M.: Lithium absorption: implications for sustained lithium preparations. Lancet 1/8319, 306 (1983)

(7) Ereshefsky, L., Saklad, S. R., Jann, M. W., Davis, Ch. M., Richards, A., Seidel, D. R.: Future of depot neuroleptic therapy: Pharmacokinetic and pharmacodynamic approaches. J. Clin. Psychiatry 45, 50–59 (1984)

(8) Famaey, J. P.: Correlation plasma levels, NSAID and therapeutic response. Clin. Rheumatol. 4, 124–132 (1985)

(9) Frenkel, E. P., McCall, M. S., Douglas, C. G., Eisenberg, S.: Fecal blood loss following aspirin and coated aspirin microspherule administration. J. Clin. Pharmacol. 8, 347–351 (1968)

(10) Gundert-Remy, U., Hildebrandt, R.: Absolute Bioverfügbarkeit einer Retard-Formulierung aus Theophyllin, Proxyphyllin und Diprophyllin nach einmaliger Gabe. In: D. Nolte, G. Krejci (eds), Methylxanthine bei obstruktiven Atemwegserkrankungen, Du-strie-Verlag Dr. Karl Feistle, München-Deisenhofen, pp 70–88 (1984)

(11) Harron, D. W. G., Shanks, R. G.: Slow release beta-adrenoceptor blocking drugs. J. R. Coll. Physicians London 17/2, 126–132 (1983)

(12) Hendeles, L., Jufrate, R. P., Weinberger, M.: A clinical and pharmacokinetic basis for the selection and use of slow release theophylline products. Clin. Pharmacokin. 9, 95–135 (1984)

(13) Kaarela, K., Lektinen, K., Mäkisara, P., Holtinen, K., Lamminsivu, U., Gordin, A.: Pharmacokinetics and tolerance of slow-release indomethacin tablets in rheumatoid arthritis. Eur. J. Clin. Pharmacol. 23, 349–351 (1982)

(14) Kleinbloesem, C. H., van Brummelen, F., van de Linde, J. A., Voogel, B. J., Breimer, D. D.: Nifedipine: Kinetics and dynamics in healthy subjects. Clin. Pharm. Ther. 35, 742–749 (1984)

(15) Kleinbloesem, C. H., van Brummelen, R., Danhof, M., Faber, H., Urquart, J., Breimer, D. D.: Rate of increase in the plasma concentration of nifedipine as a major determinant of its hemodynamic effects in humans. Clin. Pharm. Ther. 41, 26–30 (1987)

(16) Loew, D., Barkow, D., Schuster, O., Knoell, H. E.: Pharmacokinetic and pharmacodynamic study of the combination of furosemide retard and triamterene. Eur. J. Clin. Pharmacol. 26, 191–195 (1984)

(17) McAinsh, J., Baber, N. S., Smith, R., Young, J.: Pharmacokinetic and Pharmacodynamic studies with long acting propanolol. Br. J. Clin. Pharmac. 6, 115–121 (1978)

(18) Marini, J. L., Sheard, M. H.: Sustained-release lithium carbonate in a double blind study: serum lithium levels, side effects and placebo response. J. Clin. Pharmacol. 16, 276–283 (1976)

(19) Mielants, H., Veys, E. M., Verbruggen, G., Schelstraete, K.: Salicylate-induced gastrointestinal beding: Comparison between soluble buffered, enteric-coated and intravenous administration. J. Rheumatol. 6, 210–218 (1979)

(20) Perruca, E., Grimaldi, R., Gatti, G., Caravaggi, M., Crema, F., Lecchini, S., Frigo, G. M.: Pharmacokinetic and pharmacodynamic studies with a new controlled release formulation of propanolol in normal volunteers: a comparison with other commercially available formulations. Br. J. Clin. Pharmac. 18, 37–43 (1984)

(21) Saano, V., Komulainen, H.: Nifedipin induces intense nausea and vomiting in young healthy volunteers. Arch. Toxicol. Suppl. *9,* 217–218 (1986)

(22) Serlin, M. J., Orme, M. L. E., MacIver, M., Green, G. J., Sibeon, R. G., Breckenridge, A. M.: The pharmacodynamics and pharmacokinetics of conventional and long-acting propanolol in patients with moderate hypertension. Br. J. Clin. Pharmac. *15,* 519–527 (1983)

(23) Steger, W.: Treatment of hypertensive outpatients with a sustained-release dosage form of clonidine: a comparison with standard tablet therapy and long term follow-up study. Current Medical Res. op. *6,* 670–675 (1980)

(24) Tabachnik, E., Scott, P., Corréira, J.: Sustained release theophylline: a significant advance in the treatment of childhood asthma. J. Ped. *100,* 482–492 (1982)

(25) Taylor, D. R., Kinney, C. D., McDevitt, D. G.: Patient compliance with oral theophylline therapy. Br. J. Clin. Pharmacol. *17,* 15–20 (1984)

(26) Wilder, B. J., Karas, B. J., Peury, J. K., Asconape, J.: Gastrointestinal tolerance of divalproex sodium. Neurology *33,* 808–811 (1983)

II. Controlled Release Products – Pharmacokinetic Aspects

Luc P. Balant and Marianne Gex-Fabry, Geneva

Summary

The design and evaluation of controlled release drug products must take into consideration the pharmacokinetic properties of the active constituent. Among the important parameters, the apparent half-life of elimination plays a crucial role in the feasibility of such a pharmaceutical form. Other properties of the drug, such as first-pass elimination, non-linear disposition kinetics, as well as inter- and intra-individual variability must also be considered. Finally, it is often useful to consider the behaviour of the drug not only after administration of a single dose, but also at steady-state.

1. General considerations

Evaluation and subsequent interpretation of biopharmaceutical data constitute and integral part of drug product-design. At present, information derived solely from in vitro dissolution tests can rarely be extrapolated directly to the clinical situation but represents a valuable means of quality control (4, 12). Besides a few exceptions (3), there can be no substitute for in vivo studies. As drugs are designed to ameliorate or treat the symptoms of diseases, it might be argued that a quantitative measurement of pharmacological or therapeutic effect should be used to assess the performance of a new drug product. However, this approach is often fraught with difficulties, even though it has been applied successfully in some cases. When clinically evaluating a new product against a "standard" dosage form given on separate occasions, often, the biological system is insufficiently stable or the pharmacological effect cannot be measured with adequate precision. To overcome these difficulties, an indirect but more reliable and accessible index had to be found to allow quantitative evaluation of oral forms. Since in vitro dissolution tests are usually inadequate, the obvious choice is the measurement of drug in blood, plasma or, under certain conditions, in urine. These methods rely heavily on pharmacokinetics, it is thus understandable that the development of controlled release products also depends on such considerations. The aim of the present review is to underline some of the pharmacokinetic aspects important when a controlled release product is compared to an "immediate" release formulation or to another controlled release preparation.

2. Relevant pharmacokinetic parameters of the active constituent

The pharmacokinetic characteristics of the active constituent play an important role in the decision to develop a controlled release product. Unhappily, other criteria are sometimes applied, leading to controlled release formulations lacking pharmacokinetic or clinical justification.

2.1 The apparent half-life of elimination

A principle valid for most drugs is that they should be administered with sufficient frequency so that the ratio of maximum to minimum drug concentrations in blood at steady-state is less than the therapeutic range ratio (i. e. the ratio of maximum desirable over minimum desirable concentrations or ThRa), and at a dose high enough to produce effective concentrations. For a linear, one-compartment system with repetitive intravenous dosing (constant dose, constant dosing interval τ) the ratio of maximum to minimum drug concentrations in blood at steady state is given by:

$$\frac{C_{ss,\ max}}{C_{ss,\ min}} = \frac{\dfrac{D}{V} * \dfrac{1}{(1 - e^{-k*\tau})}}{\dfrac{D}{V} * \dfrac{e^{k*\tau}}{(1 - e^{-k*\tau})}} = e^{k*\tau}$$

where k is the first order elimination rate constant, D the administered dose and V the apparent volume of distribution. It follows that $e^{k*\tau}$ must be smaller or equal to the ThRa (17) or:

$$e^{k*\tau} < \text{ThRa} \quad \text{and} \quad \tau < t_{1/2} * \frac{\ln \text{ThRa}}{\ln 2}$$

As a simple rule, one may say that if the therapeutic range ratio is 2, the dosing interval should be shorter than one elimination half-life. For drugs with

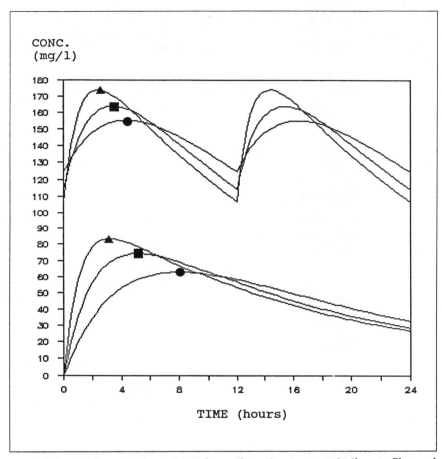

Fig. 1: Effect of decreased apparent absorption rate on concentration profiles and $C_{ss, max}/C_{ss, min}$ ratio, for a one compartment model with first-order absorption. Single dose curves are found at the bottom of the figure and steady-state profiles with 12 hours dosing intervals are represented at the top.
Absorption half-lives are 45 minutes (▲), 1.5 hours (■) and 3 hours (●). Corresponding $C_{ss, max}/C_{ss, min}$ ratios are 1.63, 1.44 and 1.25 respectively.
Elimination half-life is kept constant at 12 hours.

short half-lives (e. g. $t_{1/2} < 6h$) and low therapeutic range ratio (e. g. ThRa < 3), the proper dosing schedule requires the drug to be given unreasonably frequently.

When the drug is given orally and behaves according to a one compartment open body model with first-order absorption, the ratio of $C_{SS,max}$ over $C_{SS,min}$ is always smaller than $e^{k*\tau}$. For a given elimination rate constant, this ratio decreases as the apparent absorption rate decreases, as seen in Fig. 1. If a pharmaceutical form with an immediate release profile gives rise to a $C_{SS,max}/C_{SS,min}$ ratio which is unacceptably high, a sustained-release form may thus alleviate this problem.

The concept of a single apparent absorption rate constant describing the behaviour of the drug is based on the hypothesis that the "overall absorption

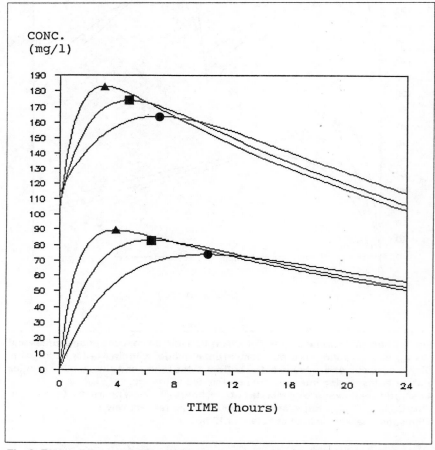

Fig. 2: Effect of decreased apparent absorption rate on concentration profiles and $C_{ss, max}/C_{ss, min}$ ratio, for a one compartment model with first-order absorption. Single dose curves are found at the bottom of the figure and steady-state profiles with 24 hours dosing intervals are represented at the top.
Absorption half-lives are 45 minutes (▲), 1.5 hours (■) and 3 hours (●). Corresponding $C_{ss, max}/C_{ss, min}$ ratios are 1.77, 1.63 and 1.44 respectively.
Elimination half-life is kept constant at 24 hours.

process" (i. e. drug release and gastro-intestinal absorption) is close to first-order. This means that the passage of drug through the gastro-intestinal wall is fast as compared to its first-order release from the pharmaceutical form. The situation seen for release patterns proportional to the square root of time is very similar to the one described here.

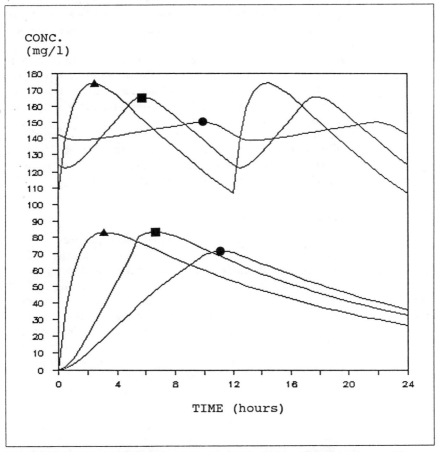

Fig. 3: Effect of zero-order release on concentration profiles and $C_{ss, max}/C_{ss, min}$ ratio, for a one compartment model with first-order absorption. Single dose curves are found at the bottom of the figure and steady-state profiles with 12 hours dosing intervals are represented at the top.
Immediate release of 1000 mg of drug (▲) is compared to zero-order release of 200 mg/h over 5 hours (■) and 100 mg/h over 10 hours (●). Corresponding $C_{ss, max}/C_{ss, min}$ ratios are 1.63, 1.34 and 1.06 respectively.
Elimination half-life is kept constant at 12 hours and true absorption half-life at 45 minutes.

It can be demonstrated that, at steady-state, the following approximations may describe $C_{SS,max}$ and $C_{SS,min}$:

$$C_{SS,max} \simeq C_{max}/[1 - EXP(-k*\tau)]$$
$$C_{SS,min} \simeq C_{min}/[1 - EXP(-k*\tau)]$$

where C_{max} and C_{min} are measured after the oral administration of the first dose and can be calculated using the Bateman function. Accordingly, the ratio of $C_{SS,max}/C_{SS,min}$ obeys more or less the same rules as after administration of a single dose if the drug kinetics is linear.

On the other hand, as seen in Fig. 2, if the apparent elimination half-life is long (e. g. $t_{1/2} > 12h$) a controlled release preparation does not usually represent a clinically useful improvement over a normal formulation if a longer action is the target parameter. For drugs with an intermediate half-life, the therapeutic range ratio is the determining factor.

When both "overall absorption" and elimination kinetics are linear processes, it may be difficult to achieve clinically relevant changes of $C_{SS,max}$ to $C_{SS,min}$ ratios. Under these conditions it may be useful to try to develop pharmaceutical forms with zero-order release properties (Fig. 3).

2.2 Absorption rates and lag-time

The difference in time between administration and detection of drug in blood or urine may be regarded as a lag-time; it may reflect delayed release of drug from the dosage form (especially enteric-coated products) and slow release or absorption coupled with insufficient sampling time. In addition, when a first-order absorption model is used to fit a curve to experimental data, an apparent lag-time often reflects non-linear gastro-intestinal absorption. Accordingly, the values calculated with pharmacokinetic models incorporating a lag-time and a first-order or zero-order absorption rate constant are often model-dependent and have probably little meaning. Other artefactual situations may also occur. For example, the drug may be decomposed by a first-order process within the gastro-intestinal tract. The overall rate constant for drug disappearance from the gastro-intestinal tract is then the sum of the true absorption rate and the decomposition rate constants and has the same value as the apparent absorption rate constant calculated from blood data. Here, the true absorption rate constant is the product of the apparent rate constant and the fraction of the dose absorbed intact, provided that hepatic first-pass metabolism is negligible (18).

With controlled release products, drug release may become the rate-limiting step in the apparent absorption process. Usually, not more than a few concentration-time points are available during the absorption phase and the absorption process is often more complex than assumed by a single first- or zero-order input. Accordingly, the calculated apparent rate constants and lag-times have little value. For **single dose studies** it is probably a wise decision not to use these calculated absorption rate constants as rate of bioavailability, but to substitute them by the two parameters C_{max} and t_{max}, if they have been properly determined.

If the combination of release and gastro-intestinal absorption rates is truly zero-order, t_{max} will unequivocally indicate the end of the release and absorption processes as with zero-order infusions. If the overall absorption rate is first-order, no such direct relationship exists since t_{max} is a function of both absorption and excretion rates. For the one-compartment open body model with first order transfers, the following equation describes t_{max}:

$$t_{max} = [\ln(k_a / k_e)]/(k_a - k_e)$$

In reality, absorption processes of controlled release preparations are often a combination of different rate constants with some deviation from true first order.

Under **steady-state conditions,** the rate of absorption should be appreciated on the basis of the amplitude between $C_{SS,max}$ and $C_{SS,min}$ (3). One may calculate a "Percentual Peak-Trough Difference" [i.e. $= 100*(C_{SS,max} - C_{SS,min})/C_{SS,av}$] or a "Percentual Swing" [i.e. $= 100*(C_{SS,max} - C_{SS,min})/C_{SS,min}$] or other combined parameters taking into account the area under the blood concentrations vs time curves (see Steinijans, 16).

The time to reach $C_{SS,max}$ can be described for the one-compartment open body model as:

$$t_{SS,max} = [1/(k_a - k_e)] * \ln \frac{k_a[1 - EXP(-k_e*\tau)]}{k_e[1 - EXP(-k_a*\tau)]}$$

The difference between T_{max} and $T_{SS,max}$ is given by:

$$t_{max} - t_{SS,max} = [1/(k_a - k_e)]*\ln \frac{[1 - EXP(-k_a*\tau)]}{[1 - EXP(-k_e*\tau)]}$$

Since the right side of this equation is always positive, it is apparent that the maximum blood concentration occurs at an earlier time at steady-state than following a single dose. Frequently, the time at which the maximum blood concentration is observed after the first dose, t_{max}, is the time at which blood is sampled after administration of subsequent doses to assess $C_{SS,max}$. Based on mathematical principles this would not be a sound practice (7).

2.3 Multicompartmental systems

Drugs with pronounced multicompartment characteristics after oral administration often show large C_{max} to C_{min} ratios. Reduced doses may be administered at intervals considerably shorter than the elimination half-life (i.e. the "longest" half-life) in order to avoid adverse effects that are associated with

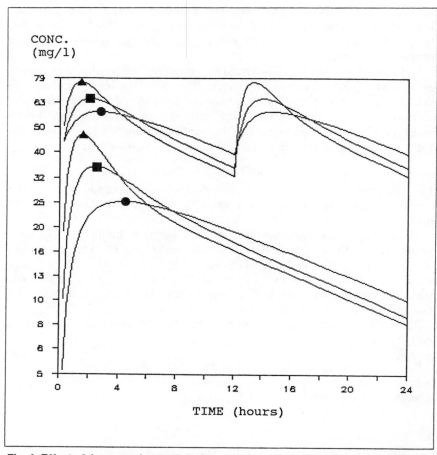

Fig. 4: Effect of decreased apparent absorption rate on concentration profiles and $C_{ss, max}/C_{ss, min}$ ratio, for a two compartment model with first-order absorption. Single dose curves are found at the bottom of the figure and steady-state profiles with 12 hours dosing intervals are represented at the top.
Absorption half-lives are 45 minutes (▲), 1.5 hours (■) and 3 hours (●). Corresponding $C_{ss, max}/C_{ss, min}$ ratios are 2.37, 1.89 and 1.48 respectively. Reduced apparent absorption rates lead to the elimination of the rapid phase decrease of the concentration versus time curve.
Elimination half-life is kept constant at 12 hours.

high drug concentrations in blood, while keeping a constant average steady-state concentration. In theory, a relatively modest reduction in the absorption rate constant of such drugs by appropriate formulation may substantially reduce the $C_{ss,max}$ to $C_{ss,min}$ ratio and may permit considerably less frequent administration of the drug. In essence, the reduced absorption rate may eliminate the "nose" of drug concentration associated with rapid absorption and slow distribution, but has little effect on the concentrations measured at the end of the dosing interval (Fig. 4). The clinical relevance of such modifications of the kinetics is, however, still an open question (see Gundert-Remy, 8).

2.4 Hepatic extraction ratio (the linear situation)

If the hepatic extraction ratio (ε) is close to one (i. e. most of the drug passing through the liver is irreversibly extracted) the systemic availability ($F = 1-\varepsilon$) is low. Generally, under these conditions, the absolute bioavailability shows great interindividual variations. Unfortunately, biopharmaceutics cannot, usually, compensate for this drawback and it is then useless to try to develop sophisticated pharmaceutical forms.

2.5 Saturable hepatic first-pass metabolism

The rate of hepatic metabolism may be limited by the amount of enzyme present in the hepatocytes or by the supply of cofactors and cosubstrates. If the drug concentration entering the organ is increased, the rate of extraction may approach a limiting value. The rate of presentation, however, goes up in proportion to the concentration. Thus the extraction ratio decreases with higher concentrations and the fraction escaping metabolism increases. For a drug that is highly cleared by the liver, the fraction escaping metabolism may be dramatically increased on going to higher concentrations. In this case, the change from a pharmaceutical form with a rapid dissolution pattern to a controlled release formulation may markedly change the systemic availability of the drug, even if the amount passing the gastro-intestinal barrier is the same.

In this situation it is not easy to perform bioavailability studies if the two pharmaceutical forms show very different release profiles. If, on the contrary, bioequivalence is tested (which implies that both rate and amount delivered should be identical), classical protocols might be adequate. Great care must then be applied during data analysis in order to avoid erroneous conclusions due to the non-linear first-pass effect. As a matter of fact, under these conditions the drug kinetics will be linear after intravenous administration and dose-dependent after oral administration if the systemic clearance is dose-independent.

2.6 Capacity-limited clearance

Concentration dependent elimination gives rise to decreased clearance at higher concentrations if elimination occurs by enzyme-catalyzed reactions or by transport-mediated processes in the liver or kidney. The area under the curve (AUC) is then not only a non-linear function of the dose, but also of the absorption rate, and/or of the release rate from the pharmaceutical preparation.

Various mathematical models have been derived for the determination of the relative bioavailability when clearance is dose-dependent. They are, however, restricted to the case where elimination is by a single saturable process, with or without a concomitant first-order elimination pathway. The power of some of these methods of estimating relative bioavailability lies in the fact that pharmacokinetic parameters such as K_M, V_{max} or k_e need not be determined explicitly if the measurements are performed under steady-state conditions. Other methods are applicable after the administration of a single dose, but require that one of the administration routes is intravenous injection. The Michaelis-Menten parameters are then estimated and used for the calculation of the bioavailability of the oral formulation. Such a method has been applied to the determination of phenytoin bioavailability and yielded an estimate of F = 0.98 as compared to F = 0.87 when linear kinetics was assumed (9).

From a practical point of view, it has been recommended that steady-state crossover-studies comparing the two different formulations (e. g. a controlled release product versus an immediate release form) at two different dose rates should be conducted when the clearance is capacity limited. One should use one dose rate at the lower end of the recommended dosing range and a second at the high end (1). For each of the two comparisons, the "new" product should meet criteria similar to those established for drugs exhibiting linear kinetics. The AUC of the "new" and the standard formulation should be equivalent according to established criteria and the degree of fluctuation of C_{max} and C_{min} of the "new" formulation should be similar to, or less than that of the standard formulation, using the value of $(C_{max}-C_{min})/C_{av}$, where C_{av} is the average concentration at steady-state (see Skelly, 14).

2.7 Saturable protein binding

A drug exhibiting saturable plasma protein binding in the therapeutic concentration range and a low extraction ratio shows non-linear clearance, but the clearance of the unbound drug is not influenced and follows linear kinetics. Accordingly, if the total plasma concentration is used to calculate AUC, both the amount and the rate of gastro-intestinal absorption influence this parameter whereas the unbound concentrations should not create such a bias (19).

If a test preparation of such a drug has a similar in vivo release-rate but a lower bioavailability than a reference preparation given at the same dose, its administration leads to lower concentrations. However, lower concentrations are associated with higher percentage of drug in plasma bound to protein and thus lower clearance. Thus, AUC based on plasma concentrations is certainly diminished, but by a lesser fraction that the bioavailability it is employed to estimate. If the test preparation has a higher bioavailability, similar reasoning dictates that AUC is increased to an extent less than the amount of drug input. In essence, this type of non-linearity causes neither relevant underestimate nor overestimate of bioavailability by AUC if the two products are given at the same dose. When the products are studied at substantially different doses, however, the "dose-correction" tends to overestimate the apparent relative bioavailability of the drug product given at the lower dose.

3. Relevant "kinetic" parameters of the volunteers

Since bioavailability studies are conducted (by definition) in living individuals, one can hypothesize that the same healthy person may absorb and eliminate the same drug differently depending on particular conditions. The analysis of all possible factors inducing intra-individual variability are beyond the scope of this review. Accordingly, only those judged relevant for controlled release preparations are presented.

3.1 Restricted gastro-intestinal area for drug absorption

If only a limited section of the gastro-intestinal tract (e.g. the so-called absorption window) is capable of absorbing a drug, either increasing the dose or decreasing the delivery rate or decreasing the transit time decreases the absorbed fraction of the administered dose (see Möller, 11). Particularly important for drugs showing incomplete gastro-intestinal absorption already in solution, this problem should be thoroughly investigated before development of a controlled release preparation.

3.2 Effect of food

Usually, bioavailability studies are performed under fasting conditions. For sustained release preparations it has, however, been advocated that the food effect should be investigated (1). The aim of such experiments should be to determine whether a food effect is present and to define whether such an effect is a result of problems with the dosage form or with the substance itself. Usually, the condition of the test is the administration of the drug product before and/or with and/or after a high fat meal. Such an experiment may require a four way crossover design. To complicate this issue, not much information seems available whether different bioequivalent drug products show behaviour differences due to food (13, see Walter-Sack, 20).

3.3 Pharmacogenetic differences

If the metabolism of a drug is under polymorphic genetic control, one may observe altered kinetics in a given fraction of the population. Thus for the debrisoquine/sparteine phenotype, about 10% of the caucasian population may be considered as poor metabolizers (5, 6, 10). At the present time, it is not clear whether subjects phenotyped as poor metabolizers should be included in bioavailability studies with the risk of a relevant increase of the inter-individual variability, or not, with the risk of missing clinically relevant differences in drug formulation behaviour. This problem certainly warrants further investigations.

3.4 Changes in urinary pH

The renal clearance of a drug may not be constant, and large intra-individual variations might exist. Substances sensitive to this type of changes are, for example, those which are mainly excreted unchanged by the kidney and showing a strong dependence on urinary pH. Accordingly, if the bioavailability of this type of medication is determined, great care must be taken in order to keep the volunteers as close as possible to some baseline state in order to minimize intra-individual variability.

The renal clearance of many bases and acids is influenced by the pH and flow of urine. Both pH and urine flow vary continuously within and between days. The sensitivity of renal clearance to pH and flow depends on the pK_a and lipid solubility of the molecule. If bioavailability studies of such drugs are based on measuring the area under the curve (AUC), then these factors are only relevant if urinary excretion of the species measured in blood is important. On the other hand, if urinary data are used, such factors are relevant under most conditions. To obviate this problem and allow assessment of the bioavailability from urinary excretion data, it has been proposed that the urinary pH be maintained constant throughout drug elimination, acidic for bases and alkaline for acids. Unfortunately, these approaches raise the question whether the agent used to render urine acidic (e.g. ammonium chloride) or alkaline (e.g. sodium bicarbonate) affect the gastro-intestinal environment sufficiently to alter the release characteristics of the drug from the dosage form and its gastro-intestinal absorption. In addition, it is evident that these measures are both inconvenient and unphysiological.

4. Planning of bioavailability studies

4.1 Volunteer selection

As stated before, all necessary precautions (including sometimes controlled food intake before the study period) must be taken in order to minimize intraindividual variability.

In some instances, especially if a steady-state study must be performed, it is necessary to administer the drug to patients who may benefit from the therapy. Patient selection becomes then a major issue because, very often, they receive other drugs which may interfere with the kinetics or the determination of the substance in the biological fluids.

Body composition and physiology at the extremes of life span, i.e. newborns and elderly, are much different from those in healthy young adults. In both extreme groups gastric acid secretion is decreased, gastric emptying time is prolonged. The absorbing area of the gastro-intestinal tract is relatively increased in newborns, but reduced in the elderly. Accordingly, it has been advocated (1) that it is desirable to evaluate sustained release dosage forms in the anticipated typical target population(s). In particular, drugs intended for use in a pediatric population should be studied in pediatric subjects. It is evident that such requirements are not easily fulfilled, at least for two reasons. First, this would dramatically increase the number of bioavailability studies needed for each drug product. Second, ethical issues are not always easily met, in particular if this type of experiments are to be conducted in small children. As a consequence, these topics are presently still controversial and normally, young healthy volunteers are recruited as the population of first choice.

4.2 Choice of the pharmaceutical forms

Usually, a single dose two-way crossover study is performed in order to compare the "new" formulation to a "reference" form, but different situations may occur.

At an early stage of development of a new drug, it might be interesting to determine the **absolute bioavailability** of a prototype formulation. Then clearly, the reference formulation should be an intravenous bolus injection or infusion. If this is not possible, one can choose a solution or a suspension of the drug in order to calculate the **relative bioavailability.**

If a **bioequivalence** study is undertaken, the reference formulation is the one for which a clinical file does exist and has been approved by the registration authorities. It is usually not recommended to use a pharmaceutical form for which only a bioequivalence trial has been performed in comparison with a standard drug product.

For controlled release preparations it might be useful to perform a three-way crossover study comparing the new formulation to a standard controlled release product and a rapidly available form such as an intravenous or oral solution. Clearly, if the potential influence of food is also to be investigated, the experimental protocol becomes more complicated.

4.3 Single dose versus steady-state studies

It is normally required to measure blood concentrations for a minimum of 3 half-lives if the drug product is studied under **single dose administration conditions,** and the wash-out period should be more than 5 half-lives (3).

When data exist for the immediate release product establishing linear kinetics, a **steady-state study** with the controlled release product may be conducted (or should be conducted according to ref. 1). At least three trough concentrations (C_{min}) over a period equal to or greater than five times the half-life of the drug should be measured to ascertain that the volunteers are at steady-state. Concentrations over at least one dosage interval of the controlled release product should be measured in each leg of the crossover. The sustained release product should produce an AUC "equivalent" to the immediate release product and the degree of fluctuation of $(C_{max}-C_{min})/C_{av}$ for the former product should be "less" than that for the latter.

The choice between single dose or steady-state designs is given essentially by practical considerations. If the elimination half-life is very short (e. g. shorter than 2 hours) it is easier to conduct a single dose study and there is little probability that multiple dose administration would change the blood concentrations markedly.

If the elimination half-life is very long, it might be very difficult to follow the blood concentrations for the required 3 half-lives and a steady-state experiment might be much easier to perform. The main concern will, however, shift from blood sampling to regular and compliant drug intake. An additional point of concern is the possible auto-enzyme-inducing properties of the drug.

If the drug shows some degree of cumulation on multiple dosing and if the analytical method is not very sensitive, a steady-state design might be valuable. Here, as in the previous case, compliance is a crucial factor.

In addition, chronopharmacokinetic aspects must also be taken into consideration if they are clinically relevant (see Staudinger, 15).

4.4 Blood sample collection

As stated above, the blood concentration profile should be measured (if possible) for at least 3 half-lives after a single dose of the drug. Sufficient samples should be available in order to allow an acceptable estimation of C_{max}, t_{max} and the elimination rate constant used to estimate the AUC from the last measured point to infinity. For slow release formulations, the determination of t_{max} may be quite problematic if the blood concentration profile is relatively flat. On the other hand, the determination of the apparent elimination rate constant may be problematic if absorption and elimination rates are similar.

It may be useful, before starting a bioavailability or a bioequivalence study with 12 or more volunteers, to undertake a pilot experiment with two subjects with frequent blood sampling. From the blood concentration-time curve one can determine an "apparent" rate of absorption and simulate the behaviour of the drug by varying this value before deciding which are the most appropriate sampling times (13). It must also be taken into account that, under steady-state conditions, t_{max} may occur earlier than after the administration of a single dose.

If the half-life measures about 6 to 8 hours, the terminal phase of the curve occurs during the night. Great care must then be taken to allow for sufficient sampling to calculate the elimination rate constant. Under these conditions, it is not acceptable to have only points until 8 p. m. and one or two data points at 8 a. m. the next morning.

4.5 Urine sample collection

It is a well accepted procedure to use urinary data for bioavailability assessments if the drug cannot be measured in blood. It might also be advisable to collect urine if a significant amount of the drug is excreted unchanged by the kidneys. The possibility to use this type of data as a complement to the determination of the area under the curve is sometimes valuable. In order to use urinary data it is important to measure the urinary pH and volume (!) of the collected samples. As many samples as possible should be collected if data analysis is to be performed, but there are clearly natural limits to the number of samples a volunteer (even well hydrated) may produce (!).

4.6 Measurement of metabolites

Usually, it is the parent compound which is used for the determination of the kinetic parameters needed to calculate the bioavailability of a drug product. In some situations (e. g. high hepatic first-pass effect with the production of active metabolites) it might be desirable to measure also the blood concentrations of a main, active metabolite. There are, however, no general rules governing this aspect of bioavailability studies.

4.7 Racemic products

It is only quite recently that pharmacokineticists have realised that drug products containing two isomers of a substance may cause problems if nonspecific analytical methods are used. Presently, there are no recommendations on this subject.

4.8 Depot preparations

Some drugs used for the treatment of chronic situations may be administered as a depot. This is for example the case for the decanoic acid esters of some antipsychotic drugs which are administered once every 2 to 4 weeks intramuscularly as an oily suspension or solution. There are presently no satisfactory means to conduct a classical bioavailability trial with these formulations which may remain in the depot for many weeks. The extent of absorption is usually considered as complete and the rate of absorption as adequate if therapeutically active concentrations can be measured over the desired time interval.

5. Conclusions

Since the initially accepted definition of bioavailability (2), an immense body of literature has accumulated on this subject. However, as our knowledge evolves, or as new pharmaceutical technologies become available, it becomes evident that our concepts and experimental designs must take these new facts into consideration. For the time being, it seems nevertheless reasonable to postulate that sound pharmacokinetic reasoning will remain the basis on which bioavailability and bioequivalence studies should be planned, interpreted and judged. This is especially true for controlled release preparations.

Last but not least, every bioavailability study should be planned, conducted and interpreted in the context of its clinical relevance.

6. Literature

(1) Report of the Workshop on Controlled Release Dosage Forms: Issues and Controversies: Academy of Pharmaceutical Sciences, American Society for Clinical Pharmacology and Therapeutics, Drug Information Association, Food and Drug Administration. Washington D.C., (1985)

(2) American Pharmaceutical Association. The Bioavailability of Drug Products. Washington D.C., (1975)

(3) Arbeitsgemeinschaft für Pharmazeutische Verfahrenstechnik. Untersuchungen zur Bioverfügbarkeit, Bioäquivalenz. Pharm. Ind. 49, 704–707 (1987)

(4) Siewert, M.: Chapter VIII.

(5) Eichelbaum, M.: Defective oxidation of drugs: pharmacokinetic and therapeutic implications. Clin. Pharmacokin. 7, 1–22 (1982)

(6) Evans, D. A. P., Mahgoub, A., Sloan, T. P., Idle, J. R., Smith, R. L.: A family and population study of the genetic polymorphism of debrisoquine in a white British population. J. Med. Genetics 17, 102–105 (1980)

(7) Gibaldi, M., Perrier, D.: Pharmacokinetics. Marcel Dekker, Inc., New York, 494 pp. (1982)

(8) Gundert-Remy, U.: Chapter I.

(9) Jusko, W. J., Koup, J. R., Alvan, G.: Nonlinear assessment of phenytoin bioavailability. J. Pharmacokin. Biopharm. 4, 327–336 (1976)

(10) Lennard, M. S., Tucker, G. T., Wood, H. F.: The polymorphic oxidation of betaadrenoceptor antagonists. Clinical pharmacokinetic considerations. Clin. Pharmacokin. 11, 1–17 (1986)

(11) Möller, H.: Chapter IV.

(12) Nicklasson, M.: Chapter IX.

(13) Ritschel, W. A.: Methodology of bioavailability assessment. S.T.P. Pharma 3, 286–301 (1987)

(14) Skelly, J. P.: Chapter X.

(15) Staudinger, H.: Chapter V.

(16) Steinijans, V. W.: Chapter VI.

(17) Theeuwes, F., Bayne, W.: Dosage form index: An objective criterion for evaluation of controlled-release drug delivery systems. J. Phar. Sci. 66, 1388–1392 (1977)

(18) Tozer, T. N.: Pharmacokinetic principles relevant to bioavailability studies. In: Principles and Perspectives in Drug Bioavailability, J. Blanchard, R. J. Sawchuk, B. B. Brodie eds. S. Karger, Basel, pp. 120–155 (1979)

(19) Upton, R. A., Williams, R. L.: The impact of neglecting non-linear plasma-protein binding on disopyramide bioavailability studies. J. Pharmacokin. Biopharm. 14, 365–379 (1986)

(20) Walter-Sack, I.: Chapter VII.

III. Controlled Release Products: Approaches of Pharmaceutical Technology

Bernhard C. Lippold, Düsseldorf

Summary

The principles used in the design of controlled release dosage forms are diffusion barriers, drug binding, slow dissolution and osmotic control of release. In applying these principles, account must be taken of some of the features required in controlled release dosage forms, ie multiple-unit principle, complete release after about 5 h, release independent of the hydrodynamics and the environment present in the stomach and small intestine, reproducibility of manufacture and of release characteristics. The release rate may be constant or may gradually decrease (1st order, $\sqrt{t}$ kinetics). In coated dosage forms retardation is effected by polymer films, often having very low permeability coefficients, since the polymer is in its glassy state. Film permeability must therefore be raised. Where aqueous polymer dispersions are used, optimal film formation is possible only at temperatures above a threshold value – the minimum film-formation temperature (MFT). Such coatings do not function as distribution membranes. For the release of a drug from matrices containing a given dose, the total porosity (initial porosity plus porosity developing with time) is of importance, and should not be too low if 100% release is to be assured. At present there is increased interest in multiple-unit matrices. The principal rate-determining step in release from hydrocolloid controlled release dosage forms is the diffusion of the active constituent through the swollen gel, but this factor is obscured to a greater or lesser extent by convective removal from the diffusion site. There is increased interest in bioadhesive hydrocolloids (prolongation of gastric residence time) and in case II diffusion (swelling-controlled diffusion with zero-order release). A brief discussion is given of some less frequently used alternatives – ion-exchange controlled release dosage forms, slow dissolution of drug, and osmotic systems. A problem affecting many controlled release dosage forms is the relation, in the case of dissociable ionic substances, between release rate and pH value and counter-ion concentration. The excipients contributing prolonged-release effects may also have pH-dependent *properties, as illustrated in some examples. Other approaches to the optimization of controlled release dosage forms involve the residence time in the stomach. In addition to adhesive dosage forms, experiments have been conducted with floating dosage forms. In future developments there will be a further increase in efforts devoted to adjusting the release of the active constituent to parallel the level of the body's requirement.*

1. Principles and requirements

Oral controlled release dosage forms may be defined as drug dosage forms from which the active ingredient is released over a long period with the aim of prolonging its action while reducing the level of side-effects (plasma peak values or fluctuation, local side-effects). At the same time, compliance should be improved by a decrease in dosing frequency. With regard to the time at which the drug is needed (eg in the early hours of the morning in the case of angina pectoris, asthma and rheumatic diseases) a controlled release dosage form allows the dose to be taken at a more convenient time (eg the previous evening).

At the design stage, account must be taken of the physico-chemical, biopharmaceutical, pharmacokinetic and pharmacodynamic properties of the drug, and of the physiological conditions in the gastro-intestinal tract.

Controlled release dosage forms are based on the principle of providing a depot or store from which the drug may be released in a controlled manner and made available for absorption only in small quantities. From the pharmacokinetic viewpoint this depot therefore constitutes a separate compartment, and the kinetics of release from this compartment are rate-determining for absorption. The initially rapid, then slower release obtained with first order, $\sqrt{t}$ or similar kinetics is especially suitable for drugs producing a cumulative plasma level (with a steady state); in this case no additional loading dose is required (39). Zero-order release (constant release rate) is advantageous for multiple dosing without accumulation. In order to bring the plasma concentration to a plateau level, a loading dose is often needed (39).

The **principles of controlled release** have long been known (39): diffusion barriers (since the early 1950s) (69), drug binding, slow dissolution and osmotic control of release. Release should be completed after about 5 hours, so that the drug may be made available for absorption in the small intestine so far as possible quantitatively (25). (Absorption from the large intestine can be used in only a few cases [41].) Where drugs are released at a gradually decreasing rate, acidic, alkali-soluble excipients may be employed to permit complete release in the lower small intestine in order to optimize bioavailability (24).

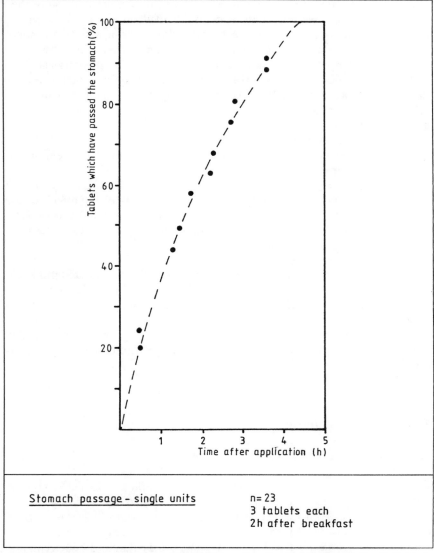

Fig. 1: Rate of clearance of intact tablets from the stomach (From Blythe, R. H. et al., ref. 5 a)

Studies performed in the 1930s and 1950s (!), extended and summarized by Nelson and Münzel (53, 55) have demonstrated the irregular and sometimes very long residence time of large dosage forms in the stomach (Fig. 1). It is only since the appearance of more recent papers by Bechgard and Davis (3,

15) that this problem has once more moved into the foreground. Since then "multiple units", multiparticulate systems (divided doses), have in general been preferred, because of their greater reliability, to "single units" or monolithic controlled release dosage forms (66). Substances having an "absorption window" are considered to be especially affected by irregular transit. This fact, and a number of other **requirements,** some arising from factors already discussed, must be taken into account in the development of controlled release dosage forms:

a. multiparticulate system;
b. slow release over a period of about 5 h;
c. release independent of the hydrodynamics (stress of the test system, motility of the GI tract);
d. release as far as possible independent of conditions in the environment of the stomach and the small intestine; food has been shown to affect release (74, 79); use can be made of pH-dependence (see above and Section 2.1);
e. reproducibility in manufacture (release) within batch and batch-to-batch (homogeneity and conformity);
f. stability of release characteristics.

If these requirements are fulfilled, making use of the above listed principles of controlled release, the dosage forms produced should provide long-lasting, reproducible blood levels exhibiting little fluctuation, and high relative bioavailability.

In the following sections the principles of controlled release are explained in more detail (with examples), new developments are presented and problems are discussed.

2. Control of release

2.1 Coated controlled release dosage forms

A development which began in the 1950s and is still continuing today was directed to the production of multiparticulate controlled release dosage forms; this development is of the greatest significance for controlling release from oral dosage forms. Highly important were two new processes which could be operated on a large technical scale: Wurster's (81) fluidized-bed technique and the production of microcapsules by coacervation (49). There were also new coating materials such as ethylcellulose (13) and methacrylic ester copolymers (35). Coatings are applied to tablets and to drug crystals, granulates and – a currently favoured alternative – pellets (diffusion pellets).

In principle, release occurs in the following stages (37, 38):
a. water, gastric juices or intestinal-tract juices penetrate the coating;

b. the drug dissolves, producing a saturated solution (c_s) if the core contains sufficient drug;

c. the drug diffuses out through the coating;

d. a constant rate of release results for so long as the concentration inside the coating remains at c_s.

Under sink conditions the release rate is given by the following expression:

$$dQ/dt = (P \cdot A / d) c \qquad\qquad\qquad\qquad \text{(Eq. 1)}$$

where:

dQ/dt	=	drug quantity released per unit time
P	=	effective permeability coefficient
A	=	area of the coating
d	=	thickness of the coating
c	=	concentration of dissolved drug inside the coating; $c = c_s$ at high drug content (37).

For drugs with molecular weights in the usual range of about 150–300, the effective permeability coefficient is dependent primarily on the coating material (40).

The actual development work involved in pharmaceutical formulation consists in adjusting the rate of release on the basis of pharmacokinetic and pharmacodynamic principles (19, 38, 43). Since the area and thickness of the coating can be varied only over a limited range, its permeability coefficient is of prime importance (43).

In general, the coating materials used – cellulose and polymethacrylate derivatives – have too low a level of permeability (37, 43, 45), and also have the disadvantage of brittleness.

The important parameters for the diffusion resistance of polymers are (40):

a. The energy of binding between neighbouring polymer chains; in amorphous polymers below the glass-transition temperature Tg this leads to the freezing of segmental movement and thus to low permeability. For example, ethylcellulose (Tg = 128 °C) (67) and quaternary methacrylate-ethacrylate copolymers (Eudragit RS and RL, Tg = about 55 °C) therefore have low permeability at 37 °C. Nevertheless, it must be remembered that, polymers take up water on contact with aqueous solutions. Since water then acts as a plasticizer, the Tg falls and permeability rises.

b. The degree of crystallinity of the polymers; crystalline, nonpermeable regions reduce the permeability, as do fillers (44).

Where coatings of low permeability are used, the followings means may be employed to raise the release rates:

a. **Incomplete coating**

This method is used unknowingly or unintentionally, but is of low reproducibility.

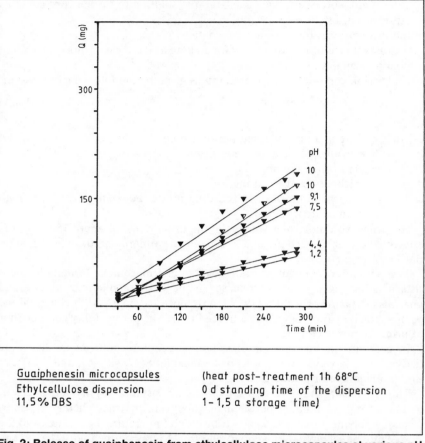

Fig. 2: Release of guaiphenesin from ethylcellulose microcapsules at various pH values

b. **Addition of plasticizers**

Plasticizers act by various mechanism (68). Firstly, they lower Tg (67). Further, they increase the uptake of water into the coating manyfold (45, 67); depending on their water solubility, they may remain in the coating (67), or be eluted (45, 67), forming micropores or macropores.

c. **Internal plasticization**

Internal plasticization may also be used to lower Tg and increase swelling by water; copolymers of methyl methacrylate and ethacrylate (Eudragit NE) have a Tg of only about 5 °C and absorb substantially more water than do PMMA homopolymers. According to the manufacturer, the permeability of such copolymers is adequate without additives.

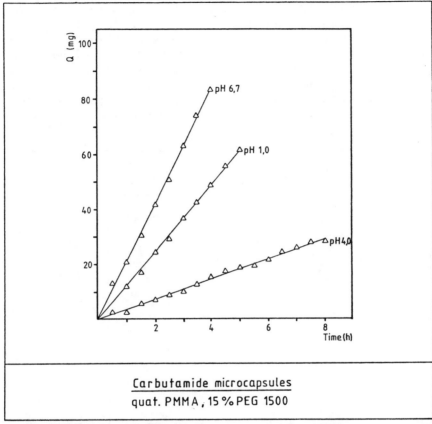

Fig. 3: Release of carbutamide from microcapsules of quaternary polymethacrylic acid/methacrylate/ethacrylate at various pH values

d. Addition of pore-formers

These include water-soluble additives such as NaCl, sucrose, cellulose derivatives or polyethylene glycols; either initially, or later during film formation (during removal of the solvent or dispersing agent), these form a disperse phase in the coating and on contact with water dissolve to leave pores (37, 42, 45, 68); also pigments which are lost from the coating at the beginning of the release process (47, 68).

The overall result is that such porous coatings, of relatively high permeability, do not behave as distribution membranes but allow both lipophilic and hydrophilic substances – including ions – to pass through. Depending on the additive used, the membranes may contain micropores (down to molecular size) or macropores, and may be homogeneous or heterogeneous (68). For this reason the release rate is a function of the total concentration c of the drug overall (undissociated and dissociated) within the coated dosage form (Eq. 1).

At the present time further developments in coatings are leading away from organic solutions of polymers, via low-solvent systems (coating emulsions) to polymer latices or pseudolatices (aqueous dispersions) (68). Formation of a continuous coating (film) is in this case more critical than in the case of the organic polymer solutions, and must be considered from the point of view of water evaporation and particle coagulation. An important factor for the for-

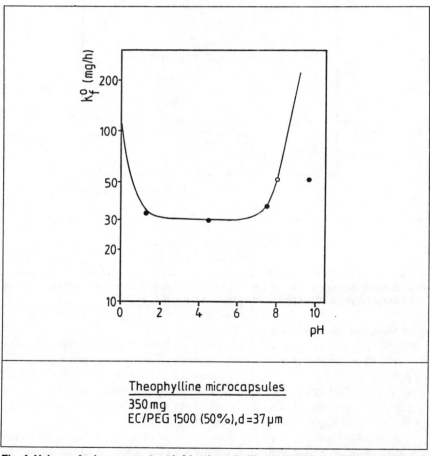

Theophylline microcapsules
350 mg
EC/PEG 1500 (50%), d =37 µm

Fig. 4: Values of release constant k_f° for theophylline from ethylcellulose microcapsules at various pH values (the line drawn through the points is the theoretical curve; a pH of 9.6 in the release medium gives a pH of only 8.1 inside the microcapsule)

mation of an optimal film coating is that the minimum film-formation temperature (MFT) (DIN, ASTM, ISO) (67, 68) should be exceeded. MFT, in turn, is critically affected by plasticizers added. Some values are (22a):

Eudragit RS 30 D (quaternary PMMA) containing 10% triacetin: 16 °C
Eudragit RS 30 D (quaternary PMMA) containing 5% triacetin: 34 °C
Eudragit RS 30 D (quaternary PMMA) containing no additive: 48 °C

Special problems arise with regard to the **pH-dependence of release.** The permeability of coatings is in general independent of pH. However, in the case of pellets with diffusion-controlled release, with coatings formed from aqueous ethylcellulose dispersions, without macropores, the permeability is observed to increase with increasing pH because of the carboxyl groups present in the ethylcellulose (67, 68); this may be a very desirable feature (Fig. 2). The pH-dependent solubility of dissociable substances may have an even more marked effect on release (Fig. 3) (37, 43, 47). However, in this system it must be remembered that the buffering effect of the drug may cause the pH inside the coating to be different from that outside (43, 47) (Fig. 4). In order to adjust the solubility to a fixed value, independent of the external pH, appropriate additives (acids, bases, buffers) may be incorporated into the core (21, 73). With reference to the dependence of the solubility, and thus the release rate, on counter-ions, see Section 2.2.

2.2 Matrices

Matrix dosage forms consist of an insoluble, in some cases porous medium (nondigestible fats, waxes and similar materials, lipophilic polymers), into which the drug and, if required, soluble additives may be incorporated (melt process, direct compression or injection-molding technique) (27, 65). In order to achieve complete release, the overall porosity ε (initial porosity resulting from included air plus porosity resulting from the dissolution of drug and additive) should be greater than 0.3. The release kinetics follow (at least approximately) Higuchi's well-known $\sqrt{t}$ law (26) (Eq. 2):

$$Q = k \cdot \sqrt{t} \qquad \text{(Eq. 2)}$$
$$Q = A \sqrt{(D \cdot \varepsilon \cdot c_s/\tau)(2 \cdot c_o - \varepsilon \cdot c_s)} \sqrt{t} \qquad \text{(Eq. 3)}$$

where:

Q = quantity of drug released
k = constant
D = diffusion coefficient of the drug in the release solution
τ = tortuosity
c_o = drug concentration in the matrix

Where the drug concentration in the matrix is relatively low ("low-load" case; $c_o < \varepsilon \cdot c_s$), however, the $\sqrt{t}$ release becomes independent of c_s and ε (10, 18, 22).

Because of the revival of interest in multiple units, more use is being made of processes leading to minimatrices:

a. matrix granulates produced, for example, by granulation with dissolved matrix-forming agents, melt granulation (50, 70);

b. matrix pellets, eg from rotor pelletizing equipment (6);

c. extrusion matrix particles with a plasticizable matrix-forming agent (20, 64), followed where necessary by spheronization (9).

Greater technical effort is required by the following products:

a. drop- or spray-congealed matrix pellets (19, 29, 51a, 61, 80);

b. matrix pellets produced by spherical agglomeration (32);

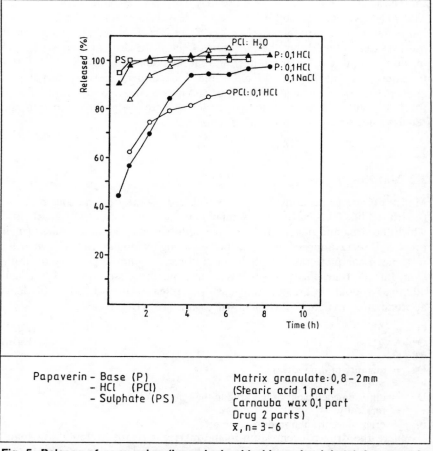

Fig. 5: Release of papaverine (base, hydrochloride and sulphate) from matrix granulates under various conditions

c. bead-polymerization matrix pellets (65);

d. matrix pellets obtained by isostatic compression (78).

We may make special reference at this point to a problem of continuous release, affecting not only matrices: the **relation between release rate and solubility product** for drugs which are salts (or acids or bases). This concerns both the adjustment of the release rate in vitro to a desired value and the behaviour in vivo. The solubility of a salt, eg a hydrochloride, in aqueous solution is not a constant; it is rather the solubility product which is constant, and the solubility therefore varies according to the concentration of chloride. This is illustrated in Fig. 5 for the release of papaverine, used as the free base, hydrochloride or sulphate, from a matrix granulate. Release of the hydrochloride into 0.1 N-HCl is markedly slower than into water, and the release of the hydrochloride into 0.1 N-HCl plus 0.1 N-NaCl is slower than into 0.1 N-HCl. The very readily soluble sulphate is practically unaffected by additives. The decision to use a specific salt must therefore be carefully considered. It must also be taken into account that in vivo the concentrations of chloride, sodium and other ions are subject to considerable variation. For example, in passing from the stomach via the duodenum to the jejunum, the chloride concentration at first increases, then decreases again.

2.3 Hydrocolloid controlled release dosage forms

Gel-forming or highly swellable substances such as cellulose derivatives, poly-acrylic acid, alginates, galactomanans, methacrylate copolymers, agar and cross-linked albumin (8, 30, 31, 33, 34, 36, 54, 56, 62, 63) have been in use as controlled release excipients since the 1960s. Quite early it became clear that release from the hydrocolloid tablets obtained proceeds substantially in accordance with the $\sqrt{t}$ law; the rate-determining step is thus the diffusion of the drug through the swollen gel matrix. In general the swelling proceeds faster than the diffusion. Some effect is exerted by the convective removal of dissolved polymer together with the drug (34). According to the extent to which release rate is affected by the hydrodynamics, this must be regarded as a more or less severe disadvantage of these products relative to coated sus-tained-release dosage forms and matrix depots, for which the release kinetics are independent of the hydrodynamics, and thus of the peristaltic process in stomach and intestine.

The production of multiple units on the basis of hydrocolloids is still at an early stage of development; processes such as bead polymerization (30) and bead formation (54) are expensive. The most promising alternative ist the use of microtablets (62).

Recently there has been increased interest in hydrocolloid depots, for two reasons:

a. possibilities of bioadhesion in the stomach;

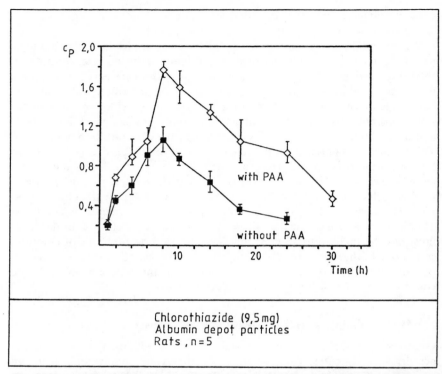

Fig. 6: Plasma levels after a dose of chlorothiazide-albumin depot particles with and without the addition of bioadhesive polyacrylic acid particles (From Longer, M. A. et al., ref. 48)

b. possibilities of zero-order release.

According to recent findings (57), anionic polymer particles, in particular, exhibit a tendency to **bioadhesion** to the mucous membrane. This effect has been exploited in order to obtain delayed transit through the stomach and intestine with a combination of cross-linked polyacrylic-acid copolymer particles with adhesive effect and drug-loaded cross-linked albumin particles. The drug used was chlorothiazide, a dibasic acid (pKa1 = 6.7; pKa2 = 9.5) having low solubility especially in acids and low bioavailability, especially at high doses and where there is a high rate of gastric emptying ("absorption window"). Tests in rats (48) showed that the bioadhesive combination remained longer in the stomach and that higher blood levels were obtained (Fig. 6). It remains for further studies to show whether gastric bioadhesion is a generally feasible route to a longer duration of action and optimized bioavailability.

Zero-order drug release from hydrocolloid depots is theoretically possible with **swelling-controlled release;** this is termed case II diffusion (1, 59). The

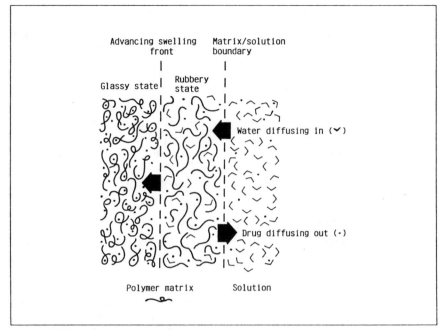

Fig. 7: Swelling-controlled release

following requirements for swelling control have been defined (Fig. 7) (59):

a. At the release temperature (37 °C) the polymer must be in the glassy state (Tg > 37 °C). Relaxation occurs on contact with water and there is gradual hydration of the polymer chains and transition into the rubbery state (Tg < 37 °C). This swelling front penetrates into the interior of the glassy polymer.

b. The inward diffusion of water must proceed at a similar rate to the advance of the swelling front and the relaxation process.

c. In comparison with the last two steps, diffusion of the drug out of the system occurs rapidly; factors important for this process are not only the properties of the drug and the polymer, but also the geometry (thickness) of the system.

Originally only cross-linked polymers were used, but recently compacts from non-cross-linked polymers have also been used (14, 51, 59, 62). This process gives approximately zero-order release, but it seems doubtful whether true case II release is achieved (51).

2.4 Dosage forms emploing erosion-controlled release

Drugs encapsulated in digestible fats are an example of conventional erosion-controlled depots (5, 17, 61). However, their use is not without its problems (17): variable enzyme activity in the gastro-intestinal tract may lead to variation in blood levels; furthermore, careful control of the fats used is required in order to guarantee reproducible release in vitro.

Eroding controlled release dosage forms have also been produced which, when lipophilic substances or high concentrations of binders are used and in the absence of excipients promoting disintegration, do not disintegrate immediately but erode from the surface inwards with the dissolution or swelling of suitable additives (58, 76, 77). Their disadvantage is their susceptibility to forced hydrodynamics during release (77) (Fig. 8).

2.5 Ion-exchange controlled release dosage forms

The use of ion-exchange-based dosage forms goes back to studies by Saunders et al. with ephedrine (12). The particulate structure of ion-exchange resins makes them suitable for processing as multiple units. Sulphonic acids are especially suitable for giving adequate delay in the release of basic drugs; release is in general too rapid from resins of the carboxylic acid type (12). The kinetics of drug release under physiological conditions are probably subject to the $\sqrt{t}$ law (matrix control); true first-order release achieved through "film control" (adhering liquid on the surface of the ion-exchange particle) can be expected more rarely (7).

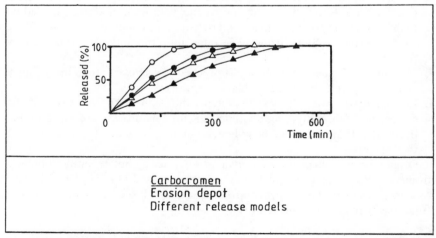

Carbocromen
Erosion depot
Different release models

Fig. 8: Release of carbocromen from an erosion depot using various release models (From Voegele, D. et al., ref. 77)

2.6 Low dissolution rate

With this technique the depot consists of undissolved and therefore nonabsorbable drug. The dissolution kinetics are rate determining for absorption. In accordance with the laws of Noyes and Whitney and of Nernst and Brunner, slow drug dissolution may be achieved to a limited extent by reducing the area (macrocrystals, eg nitrofurantoin), or employing salts of low solubility (or, in some cases, derivatives) (39).

It is less probable that a prolonged absorption will be obtained through a low saturation concentration (C_s) alone and not from a low dissolution rate. In this case the low solubility of the drug would produce slow absorption; the concentration would be maintained at saturation level by continuation of the dissolution process, assuming absorption to be very slow.

In the case of dissociable substances, factors to be taken into account are the pH-dependence of the dissolution rate and the pH range in which the concentration of the undissociated compound remains at saturation level (39, 46). The advantage that there are no problems in attaining a multiple-unit system (crystal particles) is offset by the disadvantage that the rate of dissolution decreases towards the end of the solution process (decrease in particle surface area).

2.7 Osmotic systems

Osmotic systems, whether taking the form of the elementary osmotic pump, the push-pull system or the Mini-pump are based on the interaction between an osmotically active substance, a semipermeable (ie permeable only to water) membrane and the resulting hydrostatic pressure, which induces the expulsion of drug solution thorugh a predetermined opening (16, 71, 72). In the form of the reusable Mini-pump this system is especially suitable for experimental work. Osmotic systems are classed as "therapeutic systems" (24); this term is to be regarded rather as a trade-mark, or in the context of patent law, than as describing specific dosage forms. A disadvantage is the single-unit character of osmotic systems. The factors controlling release are the properties of the membranes used, the resulting osmotic pressure and the size of the opening for egress of drug.

3. Prolongation of the residence time in the stomach

New approaches, not depending on control of the actual release rate, are aimed at prolonging the residence time of the controlled release dosage form in the stomach in order to increase the unsatisfactorily short time available for absorption. The methods include (41):

a. floating dosage forms;
b. adhesive dosage forms;
c. delaying gastric emptying.

A generally well-known example is the diazepam floating capsule (23, 52). This special capsule – which is light, floats on the stomach contents and is relatively large – remains in the stomach for several hours (in no case less than 4.3 h). It remains to be established to what extent the flotation effect – and not only the difficulty of passage through the pylorus – is of importance. Meanwhile floating-dosage forms which evolve gas, and have still greater buoyancy, have been developed (28).

Oral-adhesive-dosage forms (already mentioned in Section 2.1) have not yet emerged from the experimental stage.

The last option, delayed gastric emptying, may be achieved by the addition of fatty acid salts (25). This also causes the controlled release dosage form to remain in the stomach for a longer period, permitting considerable prolongation of release.

4. Conclusions

The methods used to confer controlled release properties on oral-dosage forms do not involve any radically new principles, but there are interesting aspects to a number of recently published techniques (special excipient properties, the effect of plasticizer in coated dosage forms, case II diffusion, gastric residence time). Moreover, problems such as the change in rate of release depending on the conditions in the gastro-intestinal environment require further studies and optimization of the pharmaceutical formulation. In an overall view, methods adopted to achieve controlled release should always be selected while bearing in mind the ultimate aim, namely to supply the drug at the rate at which it is needed. In meeting this requirement, knowledge of the pharmacokinetics and the dose-effect relationships are equally indispensable with consideration of pharmacokinetic factors and tolerance phenomena (60). We cannot ignore the fact that the dialogue between pharmacists and clinical pharmacologists provides new impetus, promotes new discoveries and brings us closer to the goal of providing the drug when and where it is needed.

5. Literature

(1) Alfrey, T., Gurnee, E. F., Lloyd, W. G.: Diffusion in Glassy Polymers. J. Polym. Sci. *C12*, 249 (1966)

(2) Bauer, K. H., Osterwald, H.: Studien über wäßrige Applikationsformen einiger synthetischer Polymere für dünndarmlösliche Filmüberzüge. Pharm. Ind. *41*, 1203 (1979)

(3) Bechgard, H.: Critical Factors Influencing Gastrointestinal Absorption – What is the Role of Pellets? Acta Pharm. Technol. *28*, 149 (1982)

(4) Benedikt, G.: Neue orale Arzneiformen und Verfahren zu ihrer Herstellung. DP 2336218 (1979)

(5) Bergauer, R., Lutz, O., Speiser, P.: Wirkstoff-Freigabe aus Fettpellets. Pharm. Ind. *39*, 1274 (1977)

(5a) Blythe, R. H., Grass, G. M., MacDonnell, D. R.: The Formulation and Evaluation of Enteric coated Aspirin Tablets. Amer. J. Pharm. *131*, 206 (1959)

(6) Bothmann, V., Mehnert, W., Frömming, K.-H.: Laboratory Scale Production of Polymer Matrix Pellets. Acta. Pharm. Technol. *34*, 17S (1988)

(7) Boyd, G. E., Adamson, A. W., Myers, L. S.: The Exchange Absorption of Ions from Aqueous Solutions by Organic Zeolithes. II. Kinetics. J. Am. Chem. Soc. *69*, 2836 (1947)

(8) Baun, D. C., Walker, G. C.: The prolonged release of caramiphen hydrochloride and atropine sulfate from compressed tablets containing carbopol[(R)] 934. Pharm. Acta Helv. *46*, 94 (1971)

(9) Briquet, F., Bossard, C., Ser. J., Duchêne, D.: Optimisation de la formulation par extrusion-sphéronisation de microgranulas matriciels à liberation prolongée. S. T. P. Pharma *2*, 986 (1986)

(10) Carstensen, J. T.: Theoretical Aspects of Polymer Matrix Systems, in Müller, B. W. (Ed.), Controlled Drug Delivery, Wissensch. Verl. Ges., Stuttgart 1987

(11) Catellani, P., Vaona, G., Plazzi, P., Colombo, P.: Compressed Matrices: Formulation and Drug Release Kinetics. Acta Pharm. Technol. *34*, 38 (1988)

(12) Chandhry, N. C., Saunders, L.: Sustained Release of Drugs from Ion Exchange Resins. J. Pharm., Pharmac. *8*, 975 (1956)

(13) Coletta, V., Rubin, H.: Wurster Coated Asperin I. Film Coating Techniques. J. Pharm. Sci. *53*, 953 (1964)

(14) Colombo, P., Gazzaniga, A., Caramella, C., Conte, U., La Manna, A.: In Vitro Programmable Zero-Order Release Drug Delivery System. Acta Pharm. Technol. *33*, 15 (1987)

(15) Davis, S. S., J.: The Design and Evaluation of controlled Release System for the Gastrointestinal Tract. J. Contr. Rel. *2*, 27 (1985)

(16) Eckenhoff, B., Theeuwes, F., Urquhart: Osmotically actuated dosage forms for rate-controlled drug delivery. J. Pharm. Techn. *5*, 35 (1981)

(17) Erni, W., Zeller, M., Piot, N.: Die Eignung von Fettpellets als Zwischenform für perorale Depotarzneiformen. Acta Pharm. Technol. *26*, 165 (1980)

(18) Fessi, H., Marty, J.-P., Puisieux, F., Carstensen, J. T.: Square Root of Time Dependence of Matrice. J. Pharm. Sci. *71*, 749 (1982)

(19) Förster, H., Lippold, B. C.: Conception of Peroral Sustained-release Dosage Forms: Calculation of Initial and Maintenance Dose with Consideration of Accumulation. Pharm. Acta Helv. *57*, 345 (1982)

(20) Grätzel von Grätz, J.: Anwendung von Extrusionsverfahren bei der Herstellung fester Arzneiformen. Acta Pharm. Technol. *34*, 42 (1988)

(21) Gruber, P., Brickl, R., Bozler, G., Stricker, H.: Neue Dipyridamol-Retardformen und Verfahren zu ihrer Herstellung. EP 0032562 (1980)

(22) Günther, J.: Dissertation, Düsseldorf, in preparation

(22a) Gunder, W.: Dissertation, Düsseldorf, in preparation

(23) Gustafson, J. H., Weissmann, L., Weinfeld, R. E., Holazo, A. A., Khoo, K.-C., Kaplan, S. A.: Clinical Bioavailability Evaluation of a Controlled Release Formulation of Diazepam. J. Pharmacokin. Biopharm. *9*, 679 (1981)

(24) Heilmann, K.: Therapeutische Systeme (Therapeutic Systems), Enke Verlag, Stuttgart 1977

(25) Heun, G. E.: Entwicklung von peroral applizierbaren Arzneiformen mit aktiv gesteuerter Gastrointestinalpassage, Dissertation Braunschweig 1987

(26) Higuchi, T.: Mechanism of sustained-Action Medication. J. Pharm. Sci. *52*, 1145 (1963)

(27) Hüttenrauch, R.: Spritzgießverfahren zur Herstellung peroraler Retardpräparate. Pharmazie *29*, 297 (1974)

(28) Ingani, H. M., Timmermanns, J., Moes, A. J.: Conception and in vivo investigation of peroral sustained release floating dosage forms with enhanced gastrointestinal transit. Int. J. Pharm. *35*, 157 (1987)

(29) John, P. M., Becker, C. H.: Surfactant effects on Spray-Congealed Formulations of Sulfaethylthiazole-Wax. J. Pharm. Sci. *57*, 584 (1968)

(30) Kala, H., Dittgen, M., Schmollack, W.: Über die Herstellung arzneistoffhaltiger Perlpolymerisate auf Polyacrylatbasis. Pharmazie *31*, 793 (1976)

(31) Kaplan, L. L.: Determination of In Vivo and In Vitro Release of Theophylline Aminoisobutanol in a Prolonged-Action System. J. Pharm. Sci. *54*, 457 (1965)

(32) Kawashima, Y., Ohno, H., Takenaka, H.: Preparation of Spherical Matrixes of Prolonged-Release Drugs from Liquid Suspension. J. Pharm. Sci. *70*, 913 (1981)

(33) Klaudianos, S.: Verfahren zur Herstellung von Retard-Tabletten auf Alginsäurebasis und Untersuchung der Wirkstoff-Freigabe. Pharm. Ind. *33*, 296 (1971); Alginat-Retard-

Tabletten-Einfluß technologischer Faktoren auf die Wirkstoff-Freigabe, I. Teil. ibid *34*, 976 (1972); Alginat-Retard-Tabletten-Einuß technologischer Faktoren auf die Wirkstoff-Freigabe, II. Teil. ibid *35*, 20 (1973)

(34) Lapidus, H., Lordi, N. G.: Some Factors Affecting the Release of a Water Soluble Drug from a Compressed Hydrophilic Matrix. J. Pharm. Sci. *55*, 840 (1966)

(35) Lehmann, K.: Acrylharzlacke zur Herstellung von Depot-Arzneiformen. Pharm. Ind. *29*, 396 (1967)

(36) Lehmann, K.: In Wasser dispergierbare, hydrophile Acrylharze mit abgestufter Permeabilität für diffusionsgesteuerte Wirkstoffabgabe aus Arzneiformen. Acta Pharm. Technol. *32*, 146 (1986)

(37) Lippold, B. C.: Solid Dosage Forms: Mechanism of Drug Release, in Polderman, J. (Ed.) Formulation and Preparation of Dosage Forms, Elsevier, Amsterdam 1977

(38) Lippold, B. C.: The Design of Pellet Systems for Controlled Drug Delivery in the GI Tract, in Breimer, D. D., Speiser, P. (Ed.), Topics in Pharmaceutical Sciences, Elsevier, Amsterdam 1983

(39) Lippold, B. C.: Biopharmazie, Wissensch. Verl. Ges., Stuttgart 1984

(40) Lippold, B. C.: Choice of Lipophilic Polymer Material for Transdermal Therapeutic Systems (TTS) and Control of Release. Pharm. Ind. *49*, 1295 (1987)

(41) Lippold, B. C.: Fortschritte und Probleme bei peroralen Retardpräparaten. Ph. Ztg. *133*, 9 (1988)

(42) Lippold, B. C., Förster, H.: Diffusion von Theophyllin durch isolierte zuschlaghaltige Ethylcellulose-Membranen. Acta Pharm. Technol. *27*, 169 (1981)

(43) Lippold, B. C., Förster, H.: Entwicklung, Herstellung und In-vitro-Testung von peroralen Depotarzneiformen mit konstanter Wirkstoffliberation am Beispiel des Theophyllins. Pharm. Ind. *44*, 735 (1982)

(44) Lippold, B. C., Kurka, P.: Füllstoffgesteuerte Freisetzung aus Suspensionsmatrices (Laminaten). Pharmazie *42*, 729 (1987)

(45) Lippold, B. C., Lippold, B. H., Sgoll, G. B.: Steuerung der Arzneistoffreisetzung aus Mikrokapseln; **1. Mitt.**, Gesetzmäßigkeiten für den Arzneistofftransport durch zuschlaghaltige lipophile Membranen. Pharm. Ind. *42*, 745 (1980)

(46) Lippold, B. H., Lichey, J. F.: Einfluß der Wasserstoffionenkonzentration auf den Membrantransport dissoziierender Arzneistoffe aus gesättigten Lösungen. Pharmazie *41*, 717 (1986)

(47) Lippold, B. H., Sgoll-Heck, G. B., Ullmann,

E.: Steuerung der Arzneistoffreisetzung aus Mikrokapseln; **2. Mitt.**, Entwicklung von Mikrokapseln mit gesteuerter Freisetzung. Acta Pharm. Technol. *27*, 121 (1981)

(48) Longer, M. A., Ch'ng, H. S., Robinson, J. R.: Bioadhesive Polymers as Platforms for Oral Controlled Drug Delivery III: Oral Delivery of Chlorothiazide Using a Bioadhesive Polymer. J. Pharm. Sci. *74*, 406 (1985)

(49) Luzzi, L. A.: Microencapsulation. J. Pharm. Sci. *59*, 1367 (1970)

(50) McTaggart, C. M., Ganley, J. A., Sickmueller, A., Walker, S. E.: The evaluation of formulation and processing conditions of a melt granulation process. Int. J. Pharm. *19*, 139 (1984)

(51) Möckel, J.: Dissertation, Düsseldorf, in preparation.

(51a) Müller, F., Laicher, A.: Untersuchungen zur In-vitro-Freisetzungskinetik aus Matrixpellets. Pharm. Ind. *45*, 189 (1982)

(52) Müller-Lissner, S. A., Will, N., Müller-Duysing, W., Heinzel, F., Blum, A. L.: Schwimmkapseln mit langsamer Wirkstoffabgabe. Dtsch. med. Wschr. *106*, 1143 (1981)

(53) Münzel, K.: Der Einfluß der Formgebung auf die Wirkung eines Arzneimittels (The effect of the shape of a dosage form on its efficacy), page 290f., Birkhäuser Verl., Basel 1966

(54) Nakano, M., Nakamura, Y., Takikawa, K., Kouketsu, M., Arita, T.: Sustained release of sulphamethizole from agar beads. J. Pharm. Pharmac. *31*, 869 (1979)

(55) Nelson, E.: Pharmacenticals for prolonged action. Clin. Pharmac. Ther. *4*, 283 (1963)

(56) Nürnberg, E., Rettig, E.: Zur Charakterisierung von Hydrokolloid-Retardtabletten, dargestellt am Beispiel "Dananden[(R)]-retard-Tabletten. Pharm. Ind. *36*, 194 (1974)

(57) Park, K., Robinson, J. R.: Bioadhesive polymers as platforms for oral-controlled drug delivery: method to study bioadhesion. Int. J. Pharm. *19*, 107 (1984)

(58) Patel, V. K., Powell, D. R.: Solid Pharmaceutical Formulations for Slow, Zero Order Release via Controlles Surface Erosion: Expanded Range. EP 0131 485 (1984)

(59) Peppas, N. A.: Swelling controlled release systems – Recent developments and applications, in Müller, B. W. (Ed.), Controlled Drug Delivery, Wissensch. Verl. Ges., Stuttgart 1987

(60) Pedersen, A. M.: Arzneimittel und Verfahren zu seiner Herstellung. DT 2414868 (1974)

(61) Ponomareff-Baumann, M., Soliva, M., Speiser, P.: Fett-Homologe als Hilfsstoffe für perorale Depot-Arzneiformen. Pharm. Acta Helv. *43*, 158 (1968)

(62) Ritschel, W. A., Gangadharan: Design and Development of a Theophylline Peroral Controlled-release Unit Dosage Forms. Pharm. Ind. *50*, 355 (1988)

(63) Salomon, J.-L., Doelker, E., Buri, P.: Sustained Release of a Water-Soluble Drug from Hydrophilic Compressed Dosage Forms. Pharm. Acta Helv. *54*, 82 (1979)

(64) Schmidt, P. C., Prochazka, J.: Über die Herstellung von Retardgranulaten durch Granulatformung. Pharm. Ind. *38*, 921 (1976)

(65) Speiser, P.: Biopharmazeutische und technische Aspekte peroraler Depot-Arzneiformen. Sci. Pharm. *37*, 14 (1969)

(66) Stanislaus, F., Huber, H. J.: Different Drug Delivery Systems in Bioavailability Studies, in Müller, B. W., Controlled Drug Delivery, Wissensch. Verl. Ges., Stuttgart 1987

(67) Sutter, B.: Wäßrige Ethylcellulosedisperionen zur Herstellung von Mikrokapseln mit gesteuerter Arzneistofffreisetzung. Dissertation, Düsseldorf 1987

(68) Sutter, B., Lippold, B. H., Lippold, B. C.: Polymerfilme als Diffusionsbarrieren für perorale Retardarzneiformen unter besonderer Berücksichtigung wäßriger Disperionen. Acta Pharm. Technol. *34*, 179 (1988)

(69) Swintosky, J. V.: Development and Design of Oral Sustained Release Dosage Forms. Ind. J. Pharm. *25*, 361 (1963)

(70) Terrier, J.-L., Touré, P., Meimoun, J., Duchêne, D., Puisieux, F.: Les comprimés XIV. Influence du Précirol[(R)] sur la libération in vitro du salicylate de sodium. Etudes per procedés de granulation et d'inclusion. Pharm. Acta. Helv. *50*, 219 (1975)

(71) Theeuwes, F.: A Physical Approach to Drug Delivery, in Borchardt, R. T., Repta, A. J., Stella, V. J., Directed Drug Delivery, Humana Press, Clifton 1985

(72) Theeuwes, F.: Elementary Osmotic Pump. J. Pharm. Sci. *64*, 1987 (1975)

(73) Thoma, K., Knott, F. X.: Verbesserung der Freisetzungskonstanz und der Verfügbarkeit von Phenothiazin-Neuroleptika sowie von Vincansin aus Resorptionsdepots mit Diffusionsüberzügen. Acta Pharm. Technol. *34*, 18S (1988)

(74) Verhoeven, J., de Boer, A. G., Junginger, H. E.: The use of microporous polymeric powders for controlled release drug delivery, in Müller, B. W. (Ed.), Controlled Drug Delivery, Wissensch. Verl. Ges., Stuttgart 1987

(75) Voegele, D.: Zur Bedeutung der Verteilungsfunktion der Freisetzungszeiten für die Galenik. Dissertation, Düsseldorf 1985

(76) Voegele, D., Schraven, E., Resag, K., Ostrowski, J.: Verfahren zur Herstellung von festen, Carbocromen-Hydrochlorid enthaltenden Präparaten. DT 2357503 (1975)

(77) Voegele, D., Brockmeier, D., Hattingberg, H. M. von, Lippold, B. C.: Die mittlere Auflösungszeit – ein Parameter zur Prüfung von Liberationsbedingungen auf Vergleichbarkeit. Acta Pharm. Technol. *29*, 167 (1983)

(78) Voegele, D., Wolff, W.: Isostatisches Verpressen, Mikrotabletten – Herstellung und Eigenschaften, APV-Kurs Neuere Erkenntnisse für die Entwicklung und Herstellung von Preßlingen (Isostatic compression, microtablets – production and properties, APV course on new findings in the development and production of tablets), Mainz 1984

(79) Wearly, L., Karim, A., Pagone, F., Streicher, J., Wickman, A.: Food-Induced Theophylline Release/Absorption Changes from Controlled-Release Formulations: A Proposed in Vitro Model. Drug Develop. Ind. Pharm. *14*, 13 (1988)

(80) Wehner, E., Voegele, D.: Mikrokugeln – Herstellung und Eigenschaften. Acta Pharm. Technol. *29*, 113 (1983)

(81) Wurster, J.: Air-Suspension Technique of Coating Drug Particles. Am. Pharm. Ass., Sci. Ed. *48*, 451 (1959)

IV. Gastro-Intestinal Absorption and Transportkinetics

Helga Möller, Frankfurt/Main

Summary

Certain information is necessary for carrying out the biopharmaceutical assessment of oral, controlled release drug products i. e. absorption kinetics of the drug substance in the different regions of the gastro-intestinal tract and the transport kinetics of the dosage form. Various techniques are used in order to assess the time-dependent absorption kinetics of drug substances; e. g. intubation techniques, endoscopic procedures and the high frequency capsule. With respect to the transport forms through the gastro-intestinal tract, gamma scintigraphy is the most common technique for monitoring the presence of dosage forms in the different regions. Both aspects – absorption and transport as a function of time – are seen as the basis for the biopharmaceutical assessment of controlled release forms.

1. Absorption

1.1 Absorption mechanisms

As early as 1940 it was pointed out that the gastro-intestinal absorption membrane is only permeable to undissociated drug substances which led to investigations on the influence exerted by the degree of dissociation, the lipid solubility of the active constituent and the pH on the site of absorption (1). The significance of ionisation and lipid solubility was demonstrated in extensive tests which support the pH distribution hypothesis (2–7). At the same time, the limits of the hypothesis were also identified since rapid intestinal absorption was detected in acidic drug substances with a pK of > 3 and basic drug substances with a pK of < 8. On the assumption that with an average intestinal pH of 6.6 the ratio of the non-ionised to the ionised proportion of an acid is 1:6000, the validity of the pH distribution hypothesis has to be revised. It was for the above reasons that the phrase a "virtual" pH was coined to indicate the pH of the intestinal epithelial cell layer. At pH 5.3, it is lower than the pH of the intestinal fluid (4).

The problematic nature of an accurate determination of the virtual pH of the intestinal epithelial cell layer is seen in the fact that in data on various values the pH is also stated at 4.5 (8), 6.1 (9) and 7 (10). This high absorption rates of weak acids observed in investigations can be explained if we assume the absorption barrier has a pH of 5. Besides the contradictory data on pH values in the absorption barrier and given the information obtained in a series of tests on weak acids such as warfarin (pK = 5.05) and acetylsalicylic acid (pK = 3.5) which reveal an absorption rate in the small intestine up to 3 times greater than that in the stomach, Benet draws the following conclusions (11):

"The nonionized form of a drug will be absorbed faster than the ionized form of the drug at any particular site in the gastrointestinal tract. However, the rate of absorption of a drug from the intestine will be greater than the gastric absorption rate of that drug even if the drug is ionized in the intestine and nonionized in the stomach."

The author is unequivocal in attributing this fact to the surface area enlarged by villi. In addition to the determination of the degree of dissociation of a substance to be absorbed, the aqueous boundary layer which is located on the epithelial cell layer and is able to influence permeation through the membrane is of great importance in the absorption process (12, 13).

The traditional concept of the pH distribution hypothesis and the relationship between the absorption and the distribution coefficients in lipid/water phases (14–16) applies mostly to lipid-soluble, apolar drug substances. Similarly, polar, hydrophilic substances such as p-amino benzoic acid (molecular weight: 137) with a pK of 4.9 and a low distribution coefficient of 0.27 (octanol/water) are absorbed well under physiological pH conditions although the substance is predominantly ionised (17–19).

Tests on an isolated, intestinal membrane of a rat showed that active transport mechanisms which are carrier-controlled by protein and sulfhydryl complexes play an important role in the absorption of p-amino benzoic acid. Evidence was also found of similar transport mechanisms through the epithelial cell layer of the intestinal rat membrane with the water-soluble antibiotics amoxcillin and cyclacillin (20).

1.2 Techniques for testing absorption

1.2.1 In vitro-tests

The influence of the degree of ionisation and the lipid/water distribution coefficient was also investigated in various in vitro tests. Distribution (21) and membrane tests (22–27) were used for this purpose. The membrane tests differ mostly in the materials of the membrane through which the drug substance penetrates when passing from the donator to the acceptor phase.

1.2.2 Animal studies

Animal studies which have become well known as intestinal perfusion methods prove suitable as in situ tests with rat intestine when investigating membrane permeation with regard to physiological criteria (28). When calculating the radius and the length of the intestinal section, time-controlled measurements of the absorbed fractions of drug substance can be made with these tests, in which the intestine of the living rat is perfused with a solution of the drug substance, by taking into account the thickness of the aqueous boundary layer, the flow rate of the perfused solution and the permeation coefficients relating to the **aqueous boundary layer** and the mucosa membrane (membrane-specific permeation coefficient).

On perfusing the rat jejunum at a rate of 0.5 ml/min, the aqueous boundary layer of the intestinal wall was measured using phenylalanin and found to have a thickness of 500 μm (29, 30) which is equal to that of a human jejunum of 630 μm at a perfusion rate of 5 ml/min and a flow rate of the boundary layer of 1.6 ml/min (31). The thickness of the aqueous boundary layer in the intestinal mucosa amounted to 950 μm on perfusion of fluid nutrients (2 ml/min) on an empty stomach at an aqueous boundary flow rate of 0.6 cm/min (32).

As regards hydrodynamics (thickness and flow rate of the aqueous boundary layer), relationships have been detected between the in situ tests and the physiological conditions in man, thus making it possible to transfer the findings from the animal tests to man (33).

The **"reserve length"** which indicates in cm the longitudinal section of the intestine in which absorption no longer takes place has been defined as the criterion for the absorption of a drug substance in the animal studies (28). On consumption of liquid nutrients, the reserve length is 225 cm in man for glucose, proteins and fat since absorption, given a total length of 325 cm (small intestine), is completed after 100 cm (33, 34). It was demonstrated by the example of corticosteroids in the animal studies that absorption is limited above the distribution coefficient of 2.5 and slows down when the flow rate of the solution of the drug substance increases. In lipid-soluble corticosteroids especially a higher membrane permeation was observed at a slower flow rate (28).

The advantages of the animal tests compared with the in vitro tests with artificial membranes can be seen in the fact that, in addition to the physicochemical properties of the drug substance, physiological function parameters are taken into account thus making it easier to transfer data to man.

1.2.3 Tests on man

Tests for bioavailability

In general, absorption is assessed using bioavailability tests by measuring the active constituent present in blood, urine or saliva. The trial design and interpretation of results for the rate (C_{max}, t_{max}) and extent of absorption (AUC) are documented in diverse guidelines (35, 36).

Detailed information on absorption kinetics can be obtained by specific computation procedures; e.g., the mass balance method. By means of numerical deconvolution (37, 38), absorption kinetics can be calculated without reference to a pharmacokinetic model as demonstrated with indomethacin (39).

Plasma concentrations as a function of time were used to assess gastrointestinal absorption subsequent to the intravenous administration of 50 mg of indomethacin as a bolus injection and after oral administration of the same dosage of indomethacin as a pH 6.8 buffered solution. The individual absorption profiles of 7 subjects are plotted on a graph in Fig. 1.

The duodenal absorption of indomethacin from a buffered solution was effected rapidly so that after 0.25 h on average approx. 50% and after 1 h not

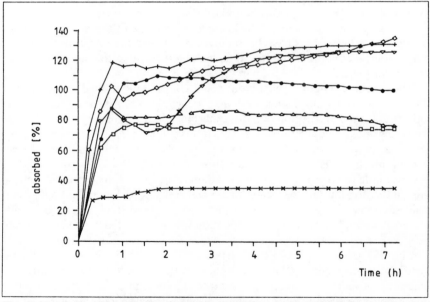

Fig. 1: Absorption kinetics of indomethacin after oral administration of a solution (50 mg of indomethacin) buffered to pH 6.8, calculated by means of deconvolution in comparison with an intravenous application (subjects 1 to 7) (From Möller, H., ref. 39).

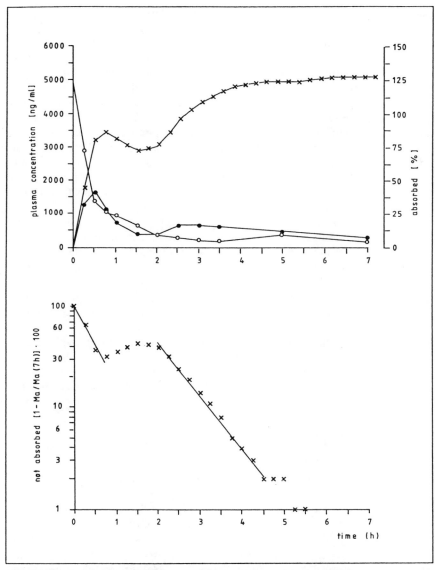

Fig. 2: Plasma concentrations and absorption kinetics of indomethacin (upper part) and bi-phasic absorption kinetics of non-absorbed indomethacin as a function of time (subject 7) (From Möller, H., ref. 39).

less than 80% of the orally administered active constituent had been absorbed.

The interpretation of the results obtained from subject 7 (Fig. 2) shows that a repeated increase in the curve of the absorption characteristics after about 2 h is due to the increase in plasma concentrations in the elimination phase of the oral solution. This suggests that enteral reabsorption takes place after emptying of the gallbladder. The extent of reabsorption can be assumed to be approximately 50% due to enterohepatic circulation. In the log/lin representation of the non-absorbed drug two processes are apparent; viz., the first phase (0–0.75 h) which takes place at a rate of 1.507 h^{-1} ($t\frac{1}{2} = 0.46$ h) and the second phase (2–4.5 h) which occurs at a roughly comparable rate constant of 1.126 h^{-1} ($t\frac{1}{2} = 0.62$ h). The first phase is attributable to absorption after oral administration (primary absorption); the second phase is due to repeated absorption from the enteral region (secondary absorption).

In so far as repeated absorption processes occur as a result of spontaneous emptying of bile into the enteral region and are detectable in the increase in plasma concentrations, the extent of reabsorption can be quantified by means of numerical deconvolution. Problems can occur however when secondary absorption processes cannot be delineated in terms of time so that reabsorption is only apparent from a continuous rise in the absorption profile.

However, a knowledge of absorption in the individual intestinal regions is especially important for the biopharmaceutical assessment of controlled release forms in which the active constituent is released during the longitudinal passage through the gastro-intestinal tract.

At present, information on time-dependent absorption obtained using the different methods discussed hereinafter is only available in the case of a few active constituents.

Intubation technique and endoscopic procedure

Using multiluminal tubes information can be obtained on absorption in the individual regions of the intestine.

The absorption of metoprolol in the jejunum and caecum was investigated by administering an infusion over 8 days and then introducing a tube through the nose on the 9th and 10th days respectively. On day 9 the distal end of the tube was positioned in the jejunum whilst being monitored radiologically and metoprolol was infused for 2.5 h. On day 10 the tube was positioned at the end of the caecum using the same technique (40). It can be inferred from the results that metoprolol has a comparable bioavailability in the jejunum and the caecum, its absolute value being approx. 40% of the intravenous injection.

Differences in the rate of absorption as a function of the intestinal region have been determined for glibenclamide by means of endoscopic tests after oral administration of a suspension (41) (Fig. 3).

On the basis of gastroscopic and coloscopic tests, mean values (AUC) of

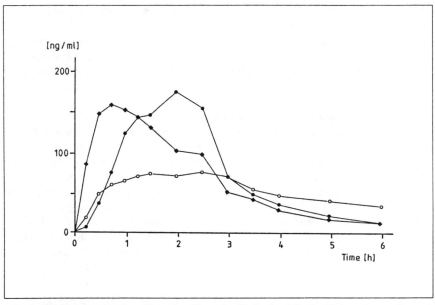

Fig. 3: The concentration-time profiles of glibenclamide for the various sites of application are shown. The median concentration curves are depicted. In 8 subjects, a suspension containing 1.75 mg of glibenclamide was instilled into the stomach (●) and duodenum (◆) in a cross over design. The same preparation was instilled into the colon (○) in a group of 6 patients. In each case the dose was placed under endoscopic control (From Bockmeier, D. et al., ref. 41).

477 ± 131 ng · h/ml (stomach), 475 ± 142 ng · h/ml (duodenum) and 486 ± 301 ng · h/ml (colon) were detected in a study of 8 subjects.

Differences in the rate of absorption became clear in the mean residence time (MT) of 2.67 ± 0.35 h (stomach), 2.42 ± 0.48 h (duodenum) and 3.55 ± 0.68 h (colon).

With comparable study designs (gastroscopic and coloscopic tests) differences were observed in the rate and extent of absorption of the diuretic, piretanide (42). Whilst comparable pharmacokinetic characteristics were calculated for the stomach (AUC: 250 ng · h/ml; MT: 1.97 h) and duodenum (243 ng · h/ml; MT: 1.51 h), distinctly divergent findings were observed for the colon (AUC: 66 ng · h/ml; MT: 3.99 h).

Using coloscopic tests evidence was also found of a bioavailability of 82% for oxprenolol in the colon which corresponds to oral administration as regards rate and extent of absorption (51).

The intubation technique makes it possible to study and quantify absorption in the proximal regions of the intestine. A drawback of this technique is that the distal intestinal regions cannot be reached and the volunteers are subject to a great deal of discomfort.

By means of endoscopic procedures such as coloscopy for example, absorption in the colon can also be studied in detail. When evaluating the test results however it should be remembered that the latter are obtained subsequent to the administration of an enema.

Artificial intestinal openings – stomata

Bieck (43) describes the possibility of assessing absorption using artificial intestinal openings (ileostomy). By comparing the amount of active constituent in the intestinal contents of patients with an ileostomy having normal faeces, information can be obtained on the absorption which has taken place.

Bieck's study team carried out tests on 2 ileostomy patients and on 7 colostomy patients in which absorption was detected by means of measurements taken from urine and intestinal contents after oral absorption of 250 mg of cliquinol. In the urine of patients with an ileostomy 11% was detected whilst in patients with a colostomy 30% was recovered as opposed to findings of 89% and 53% respectively in the intestinal contents. It can be inferred from this that more cliquinol is absorbed in the colon than in the ileum.

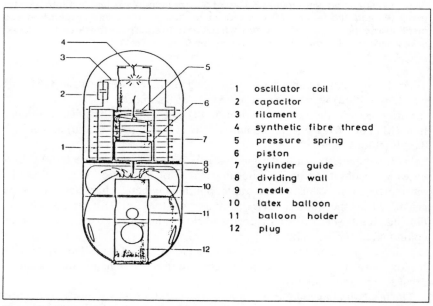

1	oscillator coil
2	capacitor
3	filament
4	synthetic fibre thread
5	pressure spring
6	piston
7	cylinder guide
8	dividing wall
9	needle
10	latex balloon
11	balloon holder
12	plug

Fig. 4: High frequency capsule (HF capsule)

High frequency capsules (HF capsules)

Reports were first made in 1981 (44) on the use of HF capsules for studying absorption in various regions of the intestine. Since then, some tests have been developed which are covered below in the form of extracts.

The HF capsule (Fig. 4) consists of a smooth plastic housing measuring 12 · 28 mm.

The device for the test material is located in one half of the capsule and consists of a mini balloon made of latex rubber which is filled by an adapter equipped with a commercial injection needle and syringe. The filled volume is about 0.7 ml. Solutions, suspensions and solids are normally suitable filling material.

The trigger mechanism is situated in the other half of the capsule and is actuated in such a way that a resonant circuit (coil and condenser) absorbs energy emitted by an external high frequency field. The absorbed energy heats the resistance wire which in turn melts through the nylon thread holding a spring under tension provided with a small needle. The water-tight core of the capsule is pierced by the force generated and the balloon is made to burst. In this way the test substance is released immediately through the available apertures in the capsule. The trigger is operated by means of a commercial 27 MHz high frequency generator and a specially designed circular antenna.

The location of the capsule in the gastro-intestinal tract and the assessment of the released drug substance on the basis of the position of the trigger mechanism is effected by X-ray examination.

Theophylline (45)

It can be deduced from present tests that theopylline shows a comparable extent of absorption in all regions of the intestine.

The HF capsules were administered to 3 subjects in the ileum and colon and their bioavailability was assessed in comparison with orally administered solutions. Whilst the extent of absorption was in all cases comparable, the absorption rate of theophylline proved to be distinctly slower in the colon (t½ abs: approx. 1.5 h).

Isosorbide-5-Mononitrate (46)

Absorption was studied in a total of 9 volunteers in the stomach (2 subjects), duodenum (2 subjects), jejunum (3 subjects) and the ascending colon (2 subjects). On administration of 20 mg of isosorbide-5-mononitrate corresponding amounts of active constituent were absorbed in the above-mentioned regions of the intestine.

Furosemide (47)

In the tests using furosemide 40 mg were administered to five volunteers in the form of a suspension in the ileocaecal region (3 subjects) and in the ascending

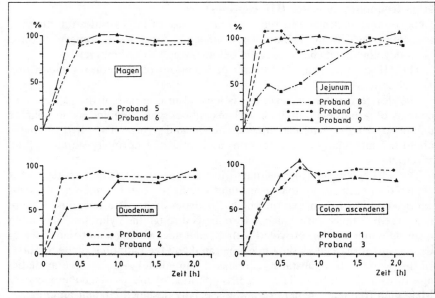

Fig. 5: Absorption of isosorbide-5-mononitrate (IS-5-MN) in various regions of the gastro-intestinal tract of healthy subjects subsequent to release from a high frequency capsule (calculated according to Wagner-Nelson) (From Wildfeuer, A. et al., ref. 46).

colon (2 subjects) by means of HF capsules. By measuring the plasma concentrations and subsequently calculating the AUC using the plasma concentrations as a function of time, it was determined, with reference to a suspension of the same dosage administered orally, that 20% of the active constituent was absorbed in the ileocaecal region as opposed to only 3% in the colon. Assuming that most absorption takes place in the duodenum and repeated, however, diminished absorption occurs in the ileocaecal region, this result accounts for a repeated increase in the plasma concentrations after approx. 11 h. Consequently, it was decided that the release of furosemide extended release forms should be timed with the transport through the gastrointestinal tract. A final conclusion however can only be drawn when the present findings have been confirmed by controlled studies using more subjects.

Allopurinol (48)

In tests on 9 subjects using allopurinol the active constituent was released in the stomach (2 subjects), duodenum (3 subjects) and mid-jejunum (2 subjects) in the form of a suspension by means of HF capsules. In the distal parts of the small intestine a distinctly reduced absorption was observed. The results point out that a maximum of 10% only of allopurinol (pka = 9.2; solubility at pH 1 to 7; approx. 50 mg/ml) is absorbed in the distal jejunum in comparison to the duodenum. Whether and to what extent the extremely low absorption in the lower jejunum can also be dependent on insufficient dissolution of the dose of 300 mg of allopurinol in the intestinal fluid must be tested by additional studies.

Indomethacin (50)

In order to determine the absorption kinetics of indomethacin in various segments of the intestine, 50 mg of indomethacin were administered to 6 subjects in the form of a suspension in the cross-over design. To assess the gastroduodenal absorption, a suspension of indomethacin (100 ml) was administered orally to the subjects who subsequently consumed 50 ml of water. Administration in the ileocaecal region and in the colon was carried out using HF capsules containing a suspension of 50 mg of indomethacin in 0.7 ml of methyl cellulose gel. Indomethacin solution administered intravenously

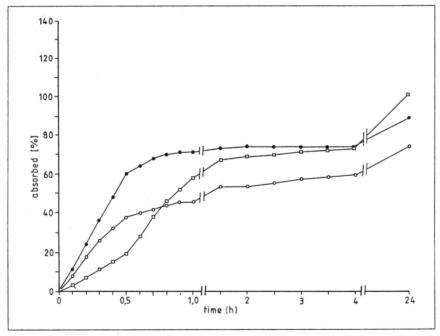

Fig. 6: Absorption kinetics of indomethacin in different regions of the gastro-intestinal tract – duodenum (□), ileocaecum (●) and colon (○), calculated by means of deconvolution of plasma concentrations. 50 mg of indomethacin were administered intraveneously (weighting function) and orally (response function) (From Möller, H., ref. 50).

served as a reference solution for the evaluation of the absolute bioavailability.

In Fig. 6 the absorption kinetics in the respective segments of the intestine calculated by numerical deconvolution are recorded as the mean values of 6 test subjects.

As a weak acid with a pk of 4.5, indomethacin is dissolved at a concentration of $4.55 \cdot 10^{-6}$ mol/l (equivalent to 0.16 mg/100 ml) at pH 3.0 and at a concentration of $7.5 \cdot 10^{-3}$ mol/l (equivalent to 269 mg/100 ml) at pH 7.5. These saturation concentrations show that the dissolution of a dose of 50 mg indomethacin depends on the pH in the gastro-intestinal tract, usually after the passage through the pylorus.

Following oral administration of the indomethacin suspension, a biphasic absorption process was affected in the first phase which took place at an average rate (ka^1) of 0.553 ± 0.41 h^{-1} (t½ = 1.25 h) by the delay in gastric emptying and the associated limited dissolution. The subsequent second phase took place on average at a rate (ka^2) of 4.103 ± 2.604 h (t½ = 0.17 h).

It can be assumed that with the second phase process the absorption in the

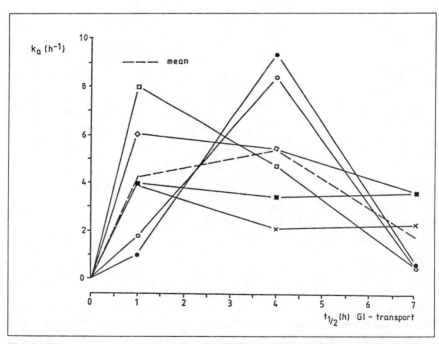

Fig. 7: Rate constants of absorption in different regions of the gastro-intestinal tract (– – – mean of subjects 1 to 6) as a function of half life (t¹/₂) of transport through the gastro-intestinal tract derived from Fig. 8.

Tab. 1: Rate and extent of absorption of indomethacin in different intestinal regions

Intestinal region	Rate k_a (h^{-1})	$t\frac{1}{2}$ (h)	AUC_{24}	Extent (%) F (24 h)	F (4 h)
Duodenum	4.103 ±2.604	0.28 ±0.23	97 ± 12	101 ± 12	73 ± 20
Ileum	5.574 ±2.826	0.16 ±0.09	85 ± 20	89 ± 24	74 ± 24
Colon	1.856 ±1.512	0.77 ±0.61	71 ± 16	75 ± 20	60 ± 26

duodenal region is not influenced by gastric conditions and, as a mean value of the 6 subjects, correlates well with the absorption in the ileocaecal region (k_a = 5.574 ± 2.826 h^{-1}; $t\frac{1}{2}$ = 0.16 h) (Fig. 7, Tab. 1).

Absorption of indomethacin in the region of the colon takes place on average k_a = 1.856 ± 1.512 h^{-1}, $t\frac{1}{2}$ = 0.77 h more slowly than in the proximal sections of the intestine as the transport through the contents of the intestine, the influence of which was very marked in some subjects, occurs as an absorption-limiting process in addition to dissolution. The delayed absorption in the colon is due to the fact that transport of the active substance to the intestinal mucosa is slowed down as a result of the thickened contents of the intestine. Consequently, it can be assumed that the rate-determining step for absorption in the colon is often represented by the transport through the intestinal contents. This is completely disregarded in coloscopy investigations because with this technique the drug is applied when the intestine is absolutely empty.

The extent of absorption in the different gastro-intestinal sections was found by area comparison with reference to intravenous administration to be 97 ± 12% for gastroduodenal absorption, 85 ± 20% for ileocaecal absorption and 71 ± 16% for absorption in the colon (Tab. 1). Absorption determined by comparison of the areas (AUC_{24}) correlates well with the amounts of drug calculated by deconvolution to have been absorbed by 24 hours (F 24 h). These are: 101 ± 12% (gastroduodenal), 89 ± 24% (ileocaecal) and 75 ± 20% (colon).

However, both methods of calculation are based on the fact that a certain amount absorbed is due to reabsorption as a result of enteral circulation and is on average between 15 and 30%, irrespective of the site of absorption. Calculation of the time and site-related extent of absorption after 4 h (F 4 h), in which secondary absorption processes were excluded, revealed an absorption of 73 ± 20% (gastro duodenal), 74 ± 24% (ileocaecal), and 60 ± 26% (colon).

Figs. 7 and 8 show a relationship between the absorption of indomethacin in

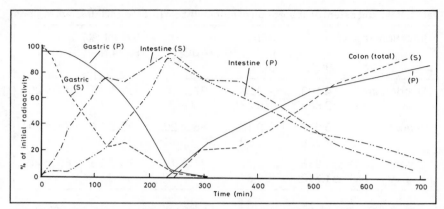

Fig. 8: Gastro-intestinal transport kinetics (mean of 6 subjects) of an indomethacin solution buffered to pH 6.8 (S) and controlled release pellets containing 50 mg of indomethacin (P) using gamma scintigraphy carried out by D. Davis, University of Nottingham.

various sections of the gastro-intestinal tract and the longitudinal transport kinetics of a solution and pellets ($\emptyset$: 0.8 to 1.2 mm).

Summing up, it may be said that in investigations on the absorption as a function of time or the intestinal segment, HF capsules represent a valuable instrument as the desired information can be obtained under natural and practical conditions. However, increased radiation exposure due to repeated radiological checks is an adverse effect. With regard to the study design, it should be pointed out that tests of this kind should be carried out with not less than 6 subjects as a high degree of variability is to be expected and fewer subjects could lead to wrong conclusions.

2. Transport kinetics of the drug products

Gastro-intestinal absorption is essentially dependent on gastric emptying and the rate of transport of the drug product through the gastro-intestinal tract whilst on the other hand, gastric emptying itself is dependent on the type of drug product and the contents of the stomach. Various methods which we have summarized (52) were used to determine gastric emptying and the rate of transport through the intestine.

2.1 Techniques for investigating transport kinetics

Extensive tagging with radiologically active material such as barium sulphate was carried out when assessing the flow rate of the stomach/intestinal contents and particular constituents of different sizes. The disadvantage of this technique is to be found in the qualitative evaluation of results and in the increase of the specific weight of the tagged material. Scintigraphy provides quantitative results in which graphs are obtained showing the chronological change of radioactivity over a larger area of the gastro-intestinal tract in a relatively short space of time. Gamma scintigraphy using radioactive nuclides which emit gamma rays is being increasingly applied in tests on the transport of the drug product during passage through the gastro-intestinal tract. During this process factors affecting transport kinetics such as type of drug product, food and position of the subject are assessed (53).

In the last 20 years scintigraphy has assumed a significant position in radiopharmacology; the field of application not being limited to diagnostics but including pharmacokinetics. In scintigraphic localisation analysis measurements of activity are carried out as functions of time and place making it possible to investigate the transportkinetics of liquid and solid dosage forms in the gastro-intestinal tract.

The radiopharmaceuticals used in scintigraphy are characterised by tagging with a radioactive nuclide which emits photon. The simultaneous emission of beta particles is of no use for measuring radiation and merely results in the patient being exposed to additonal radiation. Pure gamma emitters such as ^{99m}Tc, ^{113m}In, ^{51}Cr are therefore especially suitable for scintigraphy. Irrespective of the type of dosage form, the following requirements must be met by radioactive, tagged compounds for oral application; e. g.,
– no influence on the osmolality of the stomach contents
– no absorption and adsorption
– stability of radioactive nuclides so that no interaction occurs between the nutrients and the membrane
– miscibility with nutrients (same particle size)
– no toxicity as a result of lower radioactive doses.

2.2 Influence of the drug products

Solution and pellets
Within the scope of the investigations performed by Davis' work group at the University of Nottingham, the transport kinetics of a solution buffered to pH 6.8 (50 mg of indomethacin tagged with ^{99m}Tc) and controlled release pellets (50 mg of indomethacin, tagged with ^{99m}Tc, $\varnothing$ 0.8 to 1.2 mm, spec. weight: 1.15 g/ml) were determined via gamma scintigraphy.

The indomethacin preparations were administered immediately after a light breakfast. 90 min after administration of the drug product the subjects were allowed a cup of coffee and, 3.5 h later, a normal lunch.

Fig. 8 shows a graph of the mean radioactivity as a function of time for the

Tab. 2: Statistical comparison of the individual values of radioactivity (± SD) after oral administration of a solution buffered to pH 6.8 and retard pellets (50 mg of indomethacin).

Compound	% of the initial radioactivity in minutes (stomach)						
	20	40	50	70	125	160	235
Solution	93±8	80±17	67±18	57±13	24±16	27±17	4±6
Pellets	97±4	97±5	97±2	90±11	75±18	56±18	7±7
Significance	$p>0.1$	$0.02<$ $p<0.05$	$0.002<$ $p<0.1$	$p<0.002$	$p<0.002$	$0.02<$ $p<0.01$	$p>0.1$

solution and pellets (mean values of 6 subjects) in the compartments of the stomach, small intestine and colon. It can already be seen from the profiles of radioactivity that no statistically significant differences between the flow rate of the solution and the pellets is evident after 4 h whereas such differences are evident in the first 4 h.

On the basis of statistical comparison using the paired T-test ($p = 0.05$) the result summarized in Tab. 2 was obtained for the radioactivity values of time intervals of up to 4 h.

The time taken ($t\frac{1}{2}$) to empty the stomach of 50% of the orally administered liquid including nutritional ingredients (100 ml of indomethacin solution and approx. 350 ml of liquid in the form of breakfast) was about 85 ± 22 min. The half-life times of the liquids in other tests are in some cases lower in comparison to the findings with the indomethacin solutions, viz. approx. 12 (54), 18 (57) and 50 min respectively (56). On the whole, the differences observed are to be attributed to the differences in volume and composition of the stomach contents. Whether and to what extent the osmolality of 900 m osmol retards gastric emptying can only be subject to conjecture as present indications point to the fact that with hypertonic solutions, greater residence times are to be expected in the stomach (66).

As with the half-life times of the solutions, greater half-life times for gastric emptying were obtained for controlled release pellets than stated in literature ($t\frac{1}{2}$: 170 ± 25 min). In a study of the gastro-intestinal transport of pellets (57), an average rate of gastric emptying $t\frac{1}{2}$ of 99 ± 7 min (n = 8) has been determined by gamma scintigraphy for this divided drug product having a specific weight of 1.8 g/ml (Ø: 0.7–1.4 mm). The accelerated rate of gastric emptying in comparison with the present studies can be explained solely by the different composition of the stomach contents. This is seen in the fact that in the present study breakfast was consumed immediately before the drug product was administered as opposed to the study with the heavy pellets in which breakfast was consumed not less than 1 h before administration of the drug product. By analogy with earlier studies on patients with an ileostomy and the resultant differences in densities, slower gastric emptying is to be expected with the heavy pellets (58). However, this ist not the case when comparing the investigations carried out by Christensen et al. with the present studies (57). It could be deduced from this that both the time required for ingestion and the composition of the food have a much greater influence on gastric emptying than other factors; e.g., the specific weight of the drug product. These conclusions correspond with those from studies on capsules conducted by other authors (59).

No difference can be determined between the transport of solutions and controlled release pellets through the small intestine; the half-life times were 245 ± 85 min for the solution and 230 ± 111 min for controlled release pellets. The half-life times correlate well with the recently published studies by Christiansen et al. (57) in which rates of 246 ± 28 min (n = 5) and 204 ± 31 min (n = 8) were detected for a ^{99m}Tc-tagged solution and analogously tagged pellets respectively. From these results we can draw the conclusion that gastric emptying alone and not intestinal transport is influenced by the type of drug product used. A similar result was obtained for the transport of food which retarded gastric emptying when consumed in large amounts or in the form of a high-fat diet. In addition to this, it was proven that an increased proportion of lactulose in food does not have an effect on gastric emptying but does slow down transport in the small intestine (60). Changes in the rate of gastric emptying should only affect intestinal transport in the first 70 cm of the small intestine. Therefore, distal portions of the intestine should not be influenced. The authors describe the ileum as a buffer zone which regulates transport in the caecum (60).

As with the longitudinal, intestinal transport of the solution and controlled release pellets, no differences between the drug products are evident for the half-life times in the colon (t½ [solution] = 445 ± 82 min; t½ [pellets] = 415 ± 113 min). Christiansen et al. (57) obtained shorter half-life times in the colon with 264 ± 28 min for the solution and 304 ± 28 min for the pellets.

These discrepancies can be explained by the different intestinal motility of the subjects involved in the studies, possibly due to differences in diet. Special importance is only attached to differences of this kind in intestinal transport kinetics in as much as a reduction in absorption must be expected after 6 or even after 5 h in the biopharmaceutical evaluation of controlled release pellets containing active ingredients subjects to time-dependent absorption (55).

Indomethacin was studied in volunteers in the form of controlled release pellets with different prolongation characteristics and as a gastro-intestinal therapeutic system (GITS) (55). Results were compared with those of a pH 6.8 buffered solution of indomethacin given orally. The in vivo release, calculated by numerical deconvolution, is given as the mean value of groups of 12 and 7 subjects respectively (Fig. 9). In the upper half of Fig. 9, cumulative in

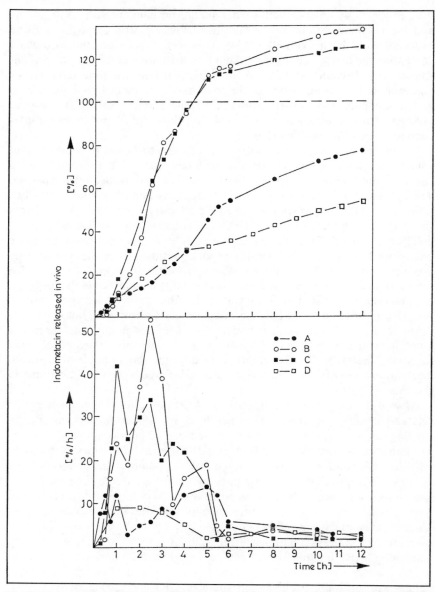

Fig. 9: In vivo release of indomethacin from pellets A, B and C (mean of 12 subjects) and gastro-intestinal therapeutic system GITS (D) (mean of 7 subjects) calculated by means of deconvolution of plasma concentration after oral administration (response function) in comparison with an oral solution (weighting function) (From Möller, H., ref. 55).

vivo release profiles of the pellets A, B and C and the gastro-intestinal therapeutic system (GITS, osmotic pump) are depicted. The fractions of the in vivo release kinetics (%/h) are given in the lower part. Although in the evaluation of the in vivo release of indomethacin from controlled release forms it must be remembered that absorption is complicated by re-absorptive processes due to enterohepatic circulation, it is nonetheless clear that the in vivo release from pellets A and from the osmotic system D is markedly prolonged and reduced compared to that from pellets B and C. The inadequate release of drug is also reflected in a bioavailability, calculated from comparison of areas under the curve (AUC), of 82% and 69%. The time-dependent absorption of indomethacin which is reduced in the colon compared to the proximal parts of the intestine by an excessive prolongation of drug release of over 6 h must also be born in mind. Therefore, optimization of the biopharmaceutical characteristics of an indomethacin controlled release form would be achieved with a multiple unit drug product giving complete release within about 5 hours.

Tablets

Enteric-coated tablets having a diameter of 5 to 7 mm pass through an empty stomach, duodenum and jejunum within 15 to 60 min and remain in the ileum for more than 200 min (61). Depending on the composition of the protective coating, disintegration of the enteric coating took between 30 and 225 min; the in vivo dissolution correlated well with the in vitro data.

However, the variability of absorption is increased with enteric-coated tablets as gastric emptying can last from a few minutes to 12 h (on average 1,5) (62). Therefore, it has proven advantageous to compress the active constituent in the form of microencapsulated tablets which disintegrate in the stomach in small particles and which behave like a "multiple dose" drug product whilst passing through the stomach and intestine. A drug product of this kind can reach the ileum/colon region after just 6 h (63).

In investigations on the bioavailability of enteric-coated tablets (Dosage: 100 mg diclofenac-sodium, weight: 210 mg, $\emptyset$: 8 mm) delayed gastric emptying of up to 3 h was even observed in the average lag time of 8 subjects (1.1 ± 0.9 h; CV = 82%) (64). Similar findings were also obtained in other studies (65) in which subjects show delayed absorption of up to 4 h both on an empty stomach and when lying down. In vivo release of every subject, calculated by numerical deconvolution of the plasma level published in (64), is plotted on a graph in Fig. 10 and is compared the in vitro release.

In tests using enteric-coated diclofenac tablets (64), the subjects were given the drug product on an empty stomach and subsequently remained supine for more than 4 h. This position is more fabourable for gastric emptying than a vertical position (67).

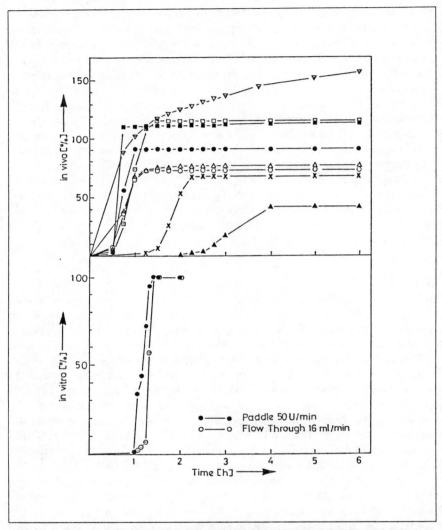

Fig. 10: In vivo-dissolution of diclofenac from enteric coated tablets (subjects 1 to 8) calculated by means of deconvolution of plasma concentration after oral administration (response function) in comparison with an oral solution (weighting function) (upper part) and in vitro-dissolution (lower part) (64).

In addition, a slowing down of gastric emptying due to the ingestion of food is avoided when the subject's stomach is empty (68). Nevertheless, in some cases a higher residence resistance time is to be expected with dimensionally stable tablets having a ∅ of 8 mm. It can be assumed that under normal living

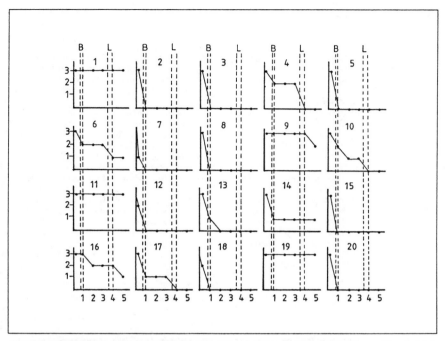

Fig. 11: Gastric emptying profile in the 20 volunteers. Abscissa: time after tablet intake (h). Ordinate: number of tablets in the stomach. B = breakfast; L = lunch (From Cortoto, A. et al., ref. 69).

conditions an average rate of gastric emptying of 0.9 ± 0.5 h is markedly increased in subjects and patients.

Corresponding to a matrix tablet in size ($\varnothing$ = 9 mm) and comparable to tablets (unit dose) as regards gastric emptying and rate of transport through the small intestine (49), osmotic pumps tagged with ^{99m}Tc behaved like gastro-intestinal therapeutic systems as half-life times of 2 to 10 h were found in 6 subjects.

As already seen in the investigations with indomethacin pellets, gastric emptying plays an important role in the characterisation of transport kinetics. The importance of gastric emptying in GITS ($\varnothing$: 8.8 mm, Thickness: 4.25 mm, Weight: 310 mg) is displayed in Fig. 11 (69).

3. Literature

(1) Travel, J.: The influence of the hydrogen ion and concentration on the absorption of alkaloids from the stomach. J. Pharmacol. *69*, 21–33 (1940)

(2) Shore, P. A. et al.: The gastric secretion of drugs. A pH partition hypothesis. J. Pharmacol. *119*, 361–369 (1950)

(3) Hogben, C. A. M. et al.: Absorption of drugs from the stomach. Part II: The human. J. Pharmacol. Exp. Ther. *120*, 540–545 (1957)

(4) Hogben, C. A. M. et al.: On the mechanism of the intestinal absorption of drugs. J. Pharmacol. *125*, 275–282 (1959)

(5) Schanker, L. S. et al.: Absorption of drugs from the stomach. Part II: The rat. J. Pharmacol. *120*, 528–539 (1957)

(6) Schanker, L. S. et al.: Absorption of drugs from the rat small intestine. J. Pharmacol. *123*, 81–88 (1958)

(7) Schanker, L. S.: Absorption of drugs from the rat colon. J. Pharmacol. *126*, 283–290 (1959)

(8) Blair, J. A. and Matty, A. J.: Acid microclimate in intestinal absorption. Clinics in Gastroenterology *3*, 183–198 (1974)

(9) Crouthamel, W. G. et al.: Drug absorption. Part IV: Influence of pH on absorption kinetics of weakly acidic drugs. J. Pharma. Sci. *60*, 1160–1163 (1971)

(10) Lucas, M. L. et al.: Direct measurement by pH microelectrode of the pH microclimate in rat proximal jejunum. Proc. Roy. Soc. London. Ser. B. *192*, 39–48 (1975)

(11) Benet, L. Z.: Biopharmaceutics as a basis for the design of drug products. In: Drug Design, published by Ariens, E. J. Volume 4, Page 1–35 Academic Press, New York (1973)

(12) Winne, D.: The influence of unstirred layers on intestinal absorption. Excerpta Medica Internat. Congress *391*, 58–64 (1975)

(13) Wilson, F. A. and Dietschy, J. M.: Characterisation of bile acid absorption across the unstirred water layer and brush border of the rat jejunum. J. Clin. Invest. *51*, 3015–3025 (1972)

(14) Houston, J. B. et al.: A re-evaluation of the importance of partition coefficients in the gastro-intestinal absorption of nutrients. J. Pharmacol. Exper. Ther. *189*, 244–254 (1974)

(15) Houston, J. B. et al.: Further studies using carbamate esters as model compounds to investigate the role of lipophilicity in the gastro-intestinal absorption of foreign compounds. J. Pharmacol. Exper. Ther. *195*, 67–72 (1975)

(16) Wood, S. G. et al.: Further consideration of the existence of an optimal partition coefficient for intestinal absorption of foreign compounds. J. Pharm. Pharmacol. *31*, 192–193 (1979)

(17) Yasuhara, M. et al.: Absorption and metabolism of p-aminobenzoic acid by rat small intestine in situ. J. Pharmacobio-Dynamics *1*, 122–131 (1978)

(18) Yasuhara, M. et al.: Absorption and metabolism of p-aminobenzoic acid by rat intestine in vitro. J. Pharmacobio-Dynamics *1*, 114–121 (1978)

(19) Yasuhara, M. et al.: Comparative studies on the absorption mechanism of p-aminobenzoic acid and p-aceto-aminobenzoic acid from the rat intestine. J. Pharmacobio-Dynamics *12*, 177–186 (1979)

(20) Kumura, T. et al.: Carrier-mediated transport systems for amonopenicillins in rat small intestine. J. Pharmacobio-Dynamics *1*, 262–267 (1979)

(21) Rosano, H. L. et al.: Mechanism of the selective flux of salts and water migration through non-aqueous liquid membranes. Phys. Chem. *65*, 1704–1708 (1961)

(22) Stricker, H.: Die in vitro-Untersuchung der "Verfügbarkeit" von Arzneistoffen. Arzneim. Forsch. *30*, 391–396 (1970)

(23) Stricker, H.: Die Arzneistoffresorption im Gastrointestinaltrakt. I. In vitro-Untersuchungen. Pharm. Ind. *33*, 157–160 (1971)

(24) Stricker, H.: Die Arzneistoffresorption im Gastrointestinaltrakt II. In vitro-Untersuchungen lipophiler Substanzen. Pharm. Ind. *35*, 13–17 (1973)

(25) Dibbern, W. H. und Scholz, G. H.: Resorptions-Modellversuche mit künstlichen Lipoidmembranen. Arzneim.-Forsch. *19*, 1140–1145 (1969)

(26) Fürst, W. und Falks M.: Arzneimittelpermeation durch künstliche Lipoidmembranen. Pharmazie *25*, 546–550 (1970)

(27) Fürst, W. und Falk, M.: Arzneimittelpermeation durch künstliche Lipoidmembranen. Pharmazie *29*, 590–593 (1974)

(28) Higuchi, W. I. et al.: Rate-limiting steps and factors in drug absorption. In: Drug absorption, published by Prescott, L. F. und Nimmo, W. S.; pp. 35–60. Adiss. Press, New York (1979)

(29) Winne, D.: Unstirred layer thickness in perfused rat jejunum in vivo. Experimentia *32*, 1278–1279 (1976)

(30) Winne, D.: Rat jejunum perfused in situ:

The effect of perfusion rate and intraluminal perfusion rate and intraluminal radius on absorption rate and effective unstirred layer thickness. Naunyn-Schmiedebergs' Archiv Pharmacol. *307*, 265–274 (1979)

(31) Read, N. W. et al.: Unstirred layer and kinetics of electrogenic glucose absorption in the human jejunum in situ. Gut *18*, 865–876 (1977)

(32) Sörgel, K. H.: Flow measurements of test meals and fasting contents in human small intestine. In: Proceeding of the International Symposium: Motility of the gastro-intestinal tract; pp. 81–96. Georg Thieme Verlag, Stuttgart (1971)

(33) Ho, N. F. H. et al.: Quantitative, mechanistic and physiologically realistic approach to the biopharmaceutical design of oral drug delivery systems. Drug. Dev. Ind. Pharm. *9*, 1111–1184 (1983)

(34) Borgström, B. et al.: Studies of intestinal digestion and absorption in the human. J. Clin. Invest. *36*, 1521–1536 (1957)

(35) Notes for Guidance of the EEC, III/573/79-EN, Investigation on Bioavailability

(36) APV-Guidelines: Studies on bioavailability and bioequivalence. Drugs made in Germany *30*, 161–166 (1987)

(37) Langenbucher, F.: Numerical convolution/deconvolution as a tool for correlating in vitro with in vivo drug availability. Pharm. Ind. *44*, 1166–1172 (1982)

(38) Langenbucher, F.: Improved understanding of convolution algorithms correlating body response with drug input. Pharm. Ind. *44*, 1275–1278 (1982)

(39) Möller, H.: Gastro-Duodenale Absorption von Indometacin Pharm. Ind. (in preparation)

(40) Godbillon, J. et al.: Investigation of Drug Absorption from the Gastro-Intestinal Tract of Man. III. metoprolol in the colon. Br. J. Clin. Pharmac. *19*, 113S–118S (1985)

(41) Brockmeier, D. et al.: Absorption of Glibenclamide from Different Sites of the Gastro-Intestinal Tract. Eur. J. Clin. Pharmac. *29*, 193–197 (1985)

(42) Brockmeier, D. et al.: The Absorption of Piretanide from the Gastro-Intestinal Tract is Site-Dependent. Eur. J. Clin. Pharmac. *30*, 79–82 (1986)

(43) Bieck, P. R.: Arzneistoffresorption aus dem menschlichen Dickdarm – neue Erkenntnisse. Acta pharma. Technol. *33*, 109–114 (1987)

(44) Zimmer, A. et al.: A novel method to study drug absorption. Proceedings of the first European Congress of Biopharmaceutics and Pharmacokinetics, Clermont Ferrand (1981)

(45) Staib, A. H. et al.: Measurement of Theophylline Absorption from Different Regions of the Gastro-Intestinal Tract Using a Remote Controlled Drug Delivery Device. Eur. J. Clin. Pharmacol. *30*, 691–697 (1986)

(46) Wildfeuer, A. et al.: Bedeutung galenischer Formen für die orale Therapie mit antianginösen Substanzen. Therapiewoche *36*, 2996–3002 (1986)

(47) Graul, E. H. et al.: Voraussetzung für die Entwicklung einer sinnvollen Retard- und Diuretikakombination. Therapiewoche *35*, 4277–4291 (1985)

(48) Schuster, O. et al.: Untersuchungen zur klinischen Pharmakokinetic von Allopurinol. Arzneim.-Forsch. *35*, 760–765 (1985)

(49) Davis, S. S.: The use of scintigraphic methods for the evaluation of drug dosage forms in the gastro-intestinal tract. Proceedings of FIP Congress (1983), Montreux

(50) Möller, H.: Pharmakokinetik, Bioverfügbarkeit und Absorptionskinetik von Indometacin in verschiedenen Abschnitten des Gastro-Intestinaltraktes. Pharma. Ind. (in preparation)

(51) Antonin, K.-H. et al.: Oxprenolol absorption in man after single bolus dosing into two segments of the colon compared with that after oral dosing. Br. J. Clin. Pharmac. *19*, 137S–142S (1985)

(52) Fell, J. T. and Digenis, G. A.: Imaging and behaviour of solid oral dosage forms in vivo. Int. J. Pharm. *22*, 1–15 (1984)

(53) Curt, N. E. et al.: The use of the gamma camera to study the gastro-intestinal transit of model drug formulations. In: Proceedings of 4th Int. Coll. Prospective Biology, Pont-à-Mousson, 1978, Karger, Basel 147–150 (1980)

(54) Clements, J. A. et al.: Kinetics of acetaminophen absorption and gastric emptying in man. Clin. Pharmacol. Ther. *24*, 420–431 (1978)

(55) Möller, H.: Biopharmaceutical Assessment of Modified Release Oral Dosage Forms. Pharma. Ind. *48*, 5, 514–519 (1986)

(56) Evans, M. A. et al.: Gastric emptying rate and the systemic availability of levodopa in the elderly parkinsonian patient. Neurology *31*, 1288–1294 (1981)

(57) Christensen, F. N. et al.: The use of gamma scintigraphy to follow the gastro-intestinal transit of pharmaceutical formulations. J. Pharm. Pharmacol. *37*, 91–95 (1985)

(57) Bechgaard, H. and Ladefoged, K.: Distribution of pellets in the gastro-intestinal tract. The influence on transit time exerted by the density or diameter of pellets. J. Pharm. Pharmacol. *30*, 690–692 (1978)

(59) Müller-Lissner, A. et al.: The effect of

specific gravity and eating on gastric empty-ing of slow-release capsules. N. Engl. J. Med. *304*, 1365 (1981)

(60) Read, N. W. et al.: Is the transit time of a meal through the small intestine related to the rate at which it leaves the stomach? Gut *28*, 824–828 (1982)

(61) Stricker, H. and Kulke, H.: Zerfall- und Pas-sage-Geschwindigkeit magensaftresistenter Tabletten im Gastrointestinaltrakt. Pharm. Ind. *43*, 1018–1021 (1981)

(62) Blythe, R. H.: The formulation and evalua-tion of sustained-release products. Drug Std. *26*, 1–11 (1958)

(63) Galeone, M. et al.: In vivo demonstration of delivery mechanisms from diversified con-trolled-release preparations. Curr. Ther. Res. *31*, 456–466 (1982)

(64) Möller, H. et al.: Bioverfügbarkeit von Dic-lonefac-Fertigarzneimittel für die orale, rektale und intramuskuläre Applikation. Pharm. Ztg. *129*, 2841–2844 (1984)

(65) Willis, J. V. et al.: The pharmacokinetics of diclofenac sodium following intravenous and oral administration. Eur. J. Clin. Pharmacol. *16*, 405–410 (1979)

(66) Read, M. W. et al.: Transit of a meal through a stomach, small intestine, and colon in nor-mal subjects and its role in the pathogenesis and diarrhoea. Gastroenterology *79*, 1276–1282 (1980)

(67) Tothill, P. et al.: The effect of posture on errors in gastric emptying measurements. Phys. Med. Biol. *25*, 1071–1077 (1980)

(68) Bates, Th. R. and Gibaldi, M.: Gastro-intestinal absorption in drugs. In: Current Concepts of the Pharmaceutical Sciences; Biopharmaceutics, published by Swarbrick, J.: Lea & Febinger, Philadelphia, PA, 57–99 (1970)

(69) Cortot, A. and Colombel, J. F.: Gastric emp-tying of OROS tablets in man. Int. J. Pharm. *22*, 321–325 (1984)

V. Chronopharmacology as a Rationale for the Development of Controlled Release Products

H. Staudinger, Konstanz

Summary

Circadian rhythms of vital functions like body temperature, heart rate, blood pressure, airway patency, absorption and secretion processes in the gastrointestinal tract and kidney function and of the serum levels of many hormones are well known. For many diseases frequently treated with sustained release formulations like bronchial asthma, rheumatoid arthritis, angina pectoris, hypertension, duodenal ulcer, chronopathological rhythms have been shown. For many drugs on the one hand chronopharmacokinetic changes – in the case of absorption also formulation dependent –, on the other hand important fluctuations in chronesthesy and chronotoxicology have been demonstrated. On this background, chronopharmacology has gained importance in recent years, it can improve treatment if used as a clinical and pharmacological rationale for the development of controlled release products. As an example the development of a chronotherapeutically optimized theophylline controlled release product for the treatment of bronchial asthma is shown.

1. Definitions

Beside the self-explanatory terms **chronopharmacology, chronopharmacokinetics,** and **chronopharmacodynamics,** the most important definitions are (8):

Amplitude (A): the measure of one half of the extent of the rhythmic change estimated by the cosine curve best fitting to the data

Chronesthesy: rhythmic (thus predictable-in-time) changes in the susceptibility or sensitivity of a target biosystem to an agent

Chronopathology: changes in an individual's biological time structure preceding coincident or following functional disorders or

	organic disease and/or time-dependent manifestation of disease
Chronotherapy:	use of treatment timed according to the stages in the sensitivity-resistance cycles of target (or non-target) tissues and organs to enhance the desired pharmacological effect and/or reduce undesirable side effects.
Frequency:	the number of cycles occurring per time unit
Mesor:	Midline Estimating Statistic of Rhythm – the value midway between highest and lowest values of the (cosine) function best fitting to the data. The M is equal to the arithmetic mean for equidistant data covering an integral number of cycles
Period:	duration of one complete cycle in a rhythmic variation
Phase:	value of a rhythmic biological variable at a certain time

2. Circadian rhythms of vital functions and hormones

Circadian rhythms of many vital functions are well known (12):
– body temperature
– heart rate
– systolic and diastolic blood pressure
– airway patency measured as airway resistance, specific conductance, FEV_1, or PEF
– absorption in the gastrointestinal tract with delayed absorption during the night of most drugs
– volume and pH of gastric juice (maximal secretion during the late evening), gastrointestinal motility, blood flow in the mesenteric vessels.
– kidney function measured as renal plasma flow and glomerular filtration rate
– pH of urine, which influences dissociation and excretion of weakly acidic or weakly alkaline drugs.

Circadian rhythms also exist for the plasma levels of most hormones such as corticosteroids, ACTH, aldosterone, insulin, STH, renin, angiotensin, adrenaline, noradrenaline, thyroxine, melatonin, endorphines and atrial natriuretic peptide.

3. Controlling of circadian rhythms, synchronizer

The most important rhythms for drug development are circadian rhythms. Light-dark cycles play obviously the most important role for synchronizing circadian rhythms (1), hormonal control seems to be mediated mainly by melatonin, a methoxyindole secreted principally by the pineal gland; it is not clear whether the retina as secondary source has only local effects or also systemic importance.

Melatonin has a high amplitude circadian rhythm with much higher plasma levels during the night, which is generated by the suprachiasmatic nucleus and entrained by the light-dark cycle. Only very bright light of more than 2500 lux stimulates the secretion of melatonin sufficiently; this is well compatible with the fact that the brightness of the light in the summer may reach 100 000 lux. Older studies conducted with light less than 500 lux suggested that social influences were more important than light-dark cycles; however, the more recent studies demonstrated clearly that the light used in the earlier studies was not bright enough. Shift work and the light conditions near the polar circuit cause a decrease of the amplitude of the melatonin rhythms and affect also other circadian rhythms.

Problems of desynchronization after sudden changes of day-/night rhythms because of shift work or as "jet lag" more pronounced with eastbound than with westbound flights are well known. The desynchronization problems associated with shift work may be solved by the adaptation of the time schedules of shift work to results of chronobiological research; however, the intercontinental air traffic – the atlantic ocean for example is crossed every day by 70 000 people – makes a drug desirable that may act as synchronizer. In the meantime, the first travellers have been treated successfully with melatonin injections.

4. Diseases with proven chronopathological rhythms

The incidence and the course of many diseases are known to have circadian rhythms, especially well known and thoroughly investigated are the circadian rhythms of pulmonary diseases like bronchial asthma. The increased incidence of nocturnal asthmatic attacks was reported by Floyer already in 1698 (7). Important impulses for the present discussion and important pathophysiological explanations were given by Barnes in 1980 (2).

Circadian rhythms of other chronic diseases are well known, too: for rheumatoid arthritis with more pain during the night and the early morning hours than during the rest of the day. Patients with angina pectoris have attacks more frequently during the night than during the day (13). On the other hand, it has been reported by several workers that myocardial infarction occurs most frequently in the morning at 10 a.m. (19). The blood pressure of patients with arterial hypertension is as in healthy subjects lower during the night than during the day. It has been shown that nifedipine lowers the blood pressure without changing the blood pressure profile over 24 hours. Pain with duodenal ulcer is more frequent during the night, it has been known since a long time that the secretion of gastric acid is markedly higher during the night (20). Tumors have been shown to have a complex system of underlying bioperiodicities, which, however, are often difficult to investigate in man (9).

5. Drugs known to exhibit chronopharmacokinetic rhythms

Studies in man and in animals have demonstrated, that rhythms of absorption, distribution, and elimination take part in chronopharmacokinetic rhythms. However, it is too early to establish general rules for the prediction of rhythms of the absorption, distribution, and elimination according to their chemical structure.

5.1 Absorption:

Drugs are generally absorbed faster after intake in the morning than after intake in the evening, i.e. C_{max} is lower and t_{max} comes later. (24). Changes of the rate of absorption may affect the extent of absorption, it has been shown for acetylsalicylic acid that the area under the curve is higher after morning than after evening intake (14). Circadian changes of the rate of absorption are likely to be increased by formulations with pH-dependent in-vitro release (3), it has been demonstrated in several instances, that the chronopharmacokinetic behaviour is not only drug – but also formulation – dependent.

In man, a slower absorption during the night has been shown for theophylline –, indomethacin –, cibenzoline –, diazepam –, amitriptiline –, propanolol – and isosorbide dinitrate – formulations.

5.2 Distribution

Only limited data are available on circadian rhythms of distribution. For cortisol, circadian changes of the volume of distribution have been shown; the volume of distribution was markedly larger at 8 a.m. compared to 4 p.m. (21).

5.3 Elimination

For valproic acid, diazepam, amitryptiline, propanolol, and hexobarbital, a higher clearance was found after evening administration compared to morning administration. The half-life of cortisol was longer after administration at 8 a.m. The data on the elimination rhythms of prednisolone (16, 6) and theophylline are equivocal (22, 24, 25).

5.3.1 Metabolization in the liver

Circadian rhythms of liver function have so far been demonstrated only in animal experiments, however, known circadian rhythms of the elimination half-lives of drugs metabolized in the liver like diazepam, amitriptyline, propanolol, and hexobarbital make circadian changes likely also in man.

Tab. 1: Chronopharmacokinetics. Drugs proven to exhibit daily variations in their pharmacokinetics in man (according to LEMMER and LABRECQUE, modified)

Cardiovascular system	Pulmonary system
Digoxin Isosorbid dinitrate Metildigoxin Propanolol Potassium chloride	Theophylline Aminophylline Terbutaline Mequitazine
Psychotropic drugs	Analgesics, antirheumatics
Diazepam Midazolam Lorazepam Amitriptyline Nortriptyline Haloperidol Lithium Diphenylhydantoine Valproic acid Hexobarbitone Mequitazine	Indomethacin Acetylsalicylic acid Aminopyrine Paracetamol Phenacetin Prednisolone
Antibiotics	Miscellaneous
Griseofulvin Sulphasymazine Sulphisomidine Ampicillin	Amphetamine Cisplatin Ethanol

5.3.2 Elimination via the kidney

It has already been mentioned, that kidney function including renal plasma flow, glomerular filtration rate, urinary volume, urinary pH and urinary electrolytes exhibit nearly dramatic changes. On the background of animal data it seems likely, that furosemide and hydrochlorothiazide are faster eliminated faster during the activity period. Urinary pH is the lowest at the end of the night and the highest around noon. Alkaline drugs like amphetamines are consequently excreted faster during the night, acid drugs sulfonamides faster during the day.

6. Chronopharmacodynamics

6.1 Chronesthesy

Best known are the differences of chronesthesy for analgesics. Reinberg found for the local anaesthetic lidocaine a 2 to 3 times longer anesthetic effect if it was administered at the skin at 4 p.m. compared to 8 a.m. Similar effects have been shown with opioids, non-opioid analgesics and endorphine levels in human blood and in rat brains.

The effect of H_1-blockers on the skin has also been shown to be related to circadian rhythms; the effect after adminstration in the morning is longer lasting, the effect after administration in the evening more pronounced.

Perhaps of the greatest relevance in current therapy is the principle of chronesthesy in the therapy of peptic ulcer disease with H_2-blockers, which is particularly in Europe nearly always performed as once-daily administration in the evening. It has been shown, that acid secretion during the night and during the following day can be inhibited with administration at 6 p.m. (17, 18).

Anticoagulation after an i.v. infusion of heparin at a constant rate over 48 hours has a circadian rhythm according to Decousus et al. (4), maxima were found shortly before midnight and in the early morning hours.

6.2 Chronotoxicity

A pronounced circadian rhythmicity of the severity of toxic effects has been shown for corticosteroids by many authors. If they are administered in the morning at the start of the activity period, the risk of adrenocortical suppression is the lowest. Administration in the evening or in the late afternoon will be followed by a greater risk of an inhibition of ACTH-secretion by the anterior lobe of the hypophysis. On the other hand, a dexamethasone-suppression test can be carried out most successful in the evening.

Probably one of the most important areas for chronotoxicological investigations is therapy of malignant disease by cytotoxic agents. As an example, less nausea, vomiting and less nephrotoxicity was found after evening administration of cis-platinum compared to morning administration (10).

Tab. 2: Chronopharmacodynamics. Drugs proven to exhibit daily variations in their effects in man (according to LEMMER and LABRECQUE, modified)

Cardiovascular system	Pulmonary system

Beta-blockers
    Acebutolol
    Atenolol
    Labetalol
    Metoprolol
    Pindolol
    Nadolol
    Oxprenolol
    Propanolol
    Sotalol
	Theophylline
	Aminophylline
	Orciprenaline
	Terbutaline
	Methylprednisolone
	Acetylcholine
	Mequitazine
	Histamine
	Ipatropium bromide

Calcium channel blockers
    Nifedipine
    Nitrendipine
    Verapamil
	Psychotropic drugs

	Diazepam Haloperidol Mequitazine
Others Glyceryl trinitrate	Analgesics, antirheumatics, local anesthetics

Isosorbide dinitrate
    Isosorbide-5-mononitrate
    Hydrochlorothiazide
    Xipamide
	Flurbiprofen
	Metamizole
	Morphine

Potassium chloride	Miscellaneous
Antihistamines	Lidocaine Doxorubin
Terfenadine Clemastine Cyproheptadine	Cisplatin Cimetidine Ranitidine
Endocrinology	Heparin Ethanol
Insulin Tolbutamide Prednisone Methylprednisolone Melatonin ACTH	Tuberculine

7. Chonoptimization of drug therapy

In a conventional development of an extended release formulation, homeostasis is anticipated despite of the fact that many body functions are known to have circadian and circannual rhythms, in a chronotherapeutical development chronopharmacological rhythms are taken into account. Most important are three areas: Rhythmicities of the disease or certain symptoms to be treated (chronopathology), pharmacokinetic and pharmacodynamic rhythmicities including chronotoxicity. For the development of an extended release formulation, circadian rhythms are most important, in some cases, especially in endocrinology, also circamensual rhythms; circannual rhythms are more important for the design and the evaluation of studies.

8. Theophylline therapy of bronchial asthma as example for a chronoptimization

It has been discussed in the previous parts that chronopathology is a part of many frequent diseases that chronopharmacokinetic rhythms have been shown for many drugs and also that chronopharmacodynamic rhythms either as rhythms of chronesthesy or as rhythms of chronotoxicity have been shown for many substances. It may therefore be expected that chronopharmocology may provide a rationale for designing a controlled release product. In the following, a classical example, the chronoptimized design of a theophylline controlled release product for the treatment of bronchial asthma will be shown.

8.1 Circadian rhythmicity of bronchial asthma

The circadian rhythmicity of bronchial asthma is well known. Dyspnoea attacks are much more common during the night, Dethlefsen and Repges (5) investigated the timing of dyspnoea attacks in 3129 still untreated, mostly asthmatic patients. Between 4 and 5 a.m. dyspnoea attacks were found 50 times more frequent than 12 hours later, between 4 and 5 p.m. Prevost et al. (22) recorded dyspnoea attacks in patients with bronchial asthma, chronic obstructive bronchitis and pulmonary emphysema. With all three diagnoses, dyspnoea attacks were shown to be most frequent during the night, the amplitude was highest with bronchial asthma. The importance of these findings is underlined by the fact that death with bronchial asthma is more common during the night (23).

Additionally to these subjective criteria, a circadian rhythmicity has also been shown for lung function parameters reflecting airway patency.

A deterioration of lung function values in the early morning hours betwen 2 and 6 a. m. has not only been shown for peak expiratory flow, which can be measured using simple equipment, but also for FEV_1, R_{aw}, and sG_{aw}. Nonspecific bronchial hyperreactivity, e. g. after challenge with histamine or acetylcholine was found to exhibit a circadian rhythm as well as reactivity after allergen provocation, e. g. with house dust mite. Recently, circadian rhythms have also been demonstrated in asthmatic patients for the concentration of inflammatory cells in broncho-alveolar lavage (15).

The circadian rhythms of lung function values and inflammatory cells are based on circadian rhythms of hormones, mediators, humoral and cellular elements of the immune system. An overview is given in Tab. 3. All rhythms are in favour of a deterioration of nocturnal airway patency.

While the clearance of theophylline does not seem to show major changes (11, 26), substantial changes of the absorption have been demonstrated. These differences may cause a markedly lower C_{max} during the night compared to the day after b. i. d. administration, which does not seem to be useful on the background of the data presented above.

An important prerequisite of a chronoptimized controlled release product is a drug release as independent as possible of pH, gastrointestinal motility, action of cholic acids and meals; this is important to provide reproducible serum profiles. For a chronoptimized theophylline formulation during the critical morning hours between 2 and 6 a. m., a reproducible plateau of high serum levels should be provided (high nocturnal excess) under the conditions of a slower absorption during the night. This should be achieved not only in

Tab. 3: Circadian rhythms of etiological factors in bronchial asthma

		time	min. / max.
Hormones	cortisol	midnight	minimum
Mediators	plasma-histamine	4 am	maximum
	total release	4 am	minimum
	antigen induced release	4 am	minimum
	PGE_2	4 am	minimum
	thromboxane	4 am	maximum
Neural factors	adrenaline	4 am	minimum
	cAMP	night	minimum
Cellular factors	lymphocytes (T_{11}, B_1)	night	maximum
	T_4	night	maximum
	Leu_8	midnight	maximum
Humoral factors	total protein	night	minimum
	IgA, IgM, IgG, IgE	night	minimum

the mean value curve but also reproducibly for each individual serum profile independent of food intake.

On the background of the slower absorption during the night, the usual b.i.d. dosing scheme seems to be inappropriate for this purpose, more suitable are either a dosing scheme with administration of ⅔ of the daily dose in the evening and administration of ⅓ in the morning or – with an even better compliance – a once-daily administration in the evening. Pronounced controlled release properties should not be the only goal for the development of a once-daily chronotherapeutic theophylline formulation, an optimized compromise between controlled release properties like low peak-trough fluctuations and a prolonged plateau coming up not too late, when the lung function values show already an improvement related to their circadian rhythm, has to be achieved.

Before the test formulation, which is used as an example, was tested in clinical trials, bioavailability, food effects with cold and warm evening meals, inter- and intraindividual reproducibility of serum theophylline profiles on different study days, b.i.d. vs. once-daily administration in the evening were tested in pharmacokinetic studies carried out in healthy volunteers.

Fig. 1 shows the typical 24 h serum theophylline profile with a prolonged plateau during the early morning hours (closed circles) vs. the profiles of a

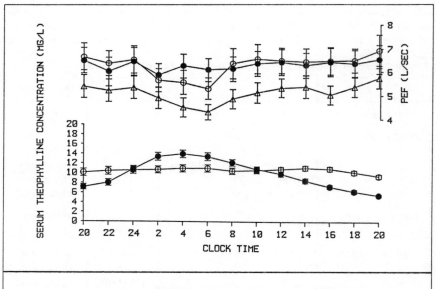

FIG. 1   MEAN +- SEM (N=20) OF SERUM THEOPHYLLINE CONCENTRATIONS AND OF PEF; INDIVIDUALIZED DOSING
Δ = PEF BASELINE   ● = TEST   O = REFERENCE

reference drug administered b.i.d. (open circles), the dose was individually titrated on the basis of the serum levels of the reference drug at 12 noon, the final dose was between 600 and 1200 mg of anhydrous theophylline. This nonmasked randomized crossover study was carried out at Herman Hospital of the University of Houston, Texas. Twenty-three of the 24 patients with bronchial asthma evaluable for the pharmacokinetic analysis were normal metabolizers of theophylline, one patient was a slow metabolizer according to the definition of the U.S. Food and Drug Administration.

8.2 Chronopharmacodynamics

The asthmatic patients taking part in this study were not selected for nocturnal symptoms or for a pre-tested early morning dip of airway patency. Measurements of PEF (peak expiratory flow), FEV_1 (forced expiratory flow in one second), $FEF_{25-75\%}$ (forced expiratory flow between 25 and 75% of the forced vital capacity) and FVC (forced vital capacity) were taken every two hours over a 24 h time span.

This study demonstrated:

1) equal efficacy over 24 hours of the chronoptimized test drug administered once daily in the evening compared to the reference drug administered b.i.d. (Fig. 1), with regard to the mesors of PEF, FEV_1, FEF, FVC and $FEV_1\%$.

2) In accordance with the chronotherapeutic concept in the critical early morning hours between 0200 and 0600 hours PEF and FEV_1 were significantly better with the test drug administered once daily in the evening than with the reference drug administered b.i.d.; moreover, this advantage was not achieved at the expense of a significantly lower PEF in the afternoon. Despite (or because) of the larger peak-trough fluctuation of serum theophylline levels with the test drug administered once daily in the evening, less circadian fluctuation of airway obstruction was observed than with the not chronoptimized reference drug administered b.i.d. This study demonstrates clearly that the chronopharmacological profile even with once-daily administration provides less fluctuation of pharmacodynamic parameters than a twice-daily administration with controlled release characteristics circumscribed as "the flatter, the better", i.e. a formulation developed without taking chronopharmacological aspects into account.

8.3 Influence of evening intake time, influence of additional medication

From a theoretical point of view, the evening intake time may be critical for a chronoptimized formulation; therefore, the clinical evaluation of this question seems to be an important step in the clinical evaluation of a chronotherapeutic theophylline controlled release product.

Bronchial obstruction cannot be stabilized by a monotherapy in most patients. The most potent bronchodilators are β_2-agonists administered by inhalation. The duration of action of most of these drugs like terbutaline, salbutamol or fenoterol is not long enough to be able to control the "early morning dip" of airway patency. Therefore, it may be suspected, that the morning dip is even more pronounced in these patients.

In the following randomized multiple crossover study in 27 outpatients, the chronoptimized test drug was administered at the three different evening intake times 6, 8, and 10 p.m. additionally to the previous therapy with β_2-agonists and inhalative corticosteroids in nearly all patients, a substantial part of the patients received also ipratropium bromide (for the complete additional medication see Tab. 4). Blood withdrawals for serum theophylline determinations and peak expiratory flow measurements were carried out every two hours in each 28 h period of measurement. The study was carried out in outpatients only hospitalized for the 28 h periods of measurements during different seasons to minimize the risk of significant periodic effects.

The pharmacodynamic results (Fig. 2) show:

1) No important differences concerning the pharmacokinetic parameters were found between the three different intake times 6, 8, and 10 p.m. It could be concluded that the evening intake time is not critical with respect to the pharmacokinetic parameters.

2) A marked, significant improvement of 24 h lung function data after adding theophylline to a modern drug therapy including inhalative β_2-agonists and corticosteroids in nearly all and inhalative anticholinergics in a substantial proportion of the treated outpatients. The mesors of the peak expiratory values did not show any significant difference.

3) During the early morning hours between 2 and 6 a.m. intake at 10 p.m. resulted in the highest nocturnal excess and the highest peak expiratory

Tab. 4: Additional medication (n = 27)

DRUG	n	%
β 2-agonists by inhalation	26	96
additionally oral β 2-agonist	1	4
additionally nasal β 2-agonist	1	4
corticosteroids by MDI	24	89
additionally oral corticosteroids	6	22
additionally nasal corticosteroids	1	4
anticholinergics by MDI	12	44
cromolyn sodium by inhalation	1	4
ketotifen	3	11

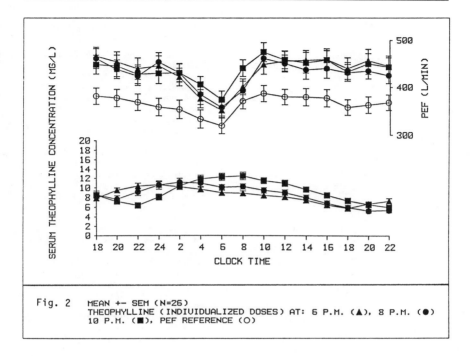

Fig. 2   MEAN +- SEM (N=26)
THEOPHYLLINE (INDIVIDUALIZED DOSES) AT: 6 P.M. (▲), 8 P.M. (●)
10 P.M. (■), PEF REFERENCE (O)

flow values. The intake at 10 p.m. may be therefore superior in patients with pronounced nocturnal problems.

4) The nocturnal peak flow between 2 and 6 o' clock a.m. improved significantly for all three intake times; however, in contrast to the previous study without additional medication, the early morning dip could not be abandoned, most likely since the efficacy of the additional medication, which did not have a chronopharmacological profile, faded already during the critical morning hours. It would be interesting to study the effect of new long acting β_2-agonists as additional medication.

The first study has proven that a chronoptimized design of a controlled release product has therapeutic advantages, the second study has demonstrated the stability of the concept with different evening intake times. The chroneffectivity may be partially disturbed by not chronoptimized additional medication, which is not an argument against the chronoptimized formulation but rather an argument against the use of not chronoptimized formulations as additional medication. In conclusion, a chronopharmacological concept should be considered more frequently for the design of controlled release formulations.

9. Literature

(1) Arendt, A. and Broadway, J.: Light and Melatonin as Zeitgebers in Man *4*, 273–282 (1987) Chronobiology International, Vol. 4, No. 2, pp. 273–282, 1987

(2) Barnes, P.: Nocturnal Asthma and Changes in Circulating Epinephrine, Histamine, and Cortisol. N. Engl. J. Med. *303*, 263–267 (1980)

(3) Coulthard, K. P., Birkett, D. J., Lines, D. R., Grgurinovich, B. J. and Grygiel, J. J.: Bioavailability and Diurnal Variation in Absorption of Sustained Release Theophylline in Asthmatic Children. Eur. J. Clin. Pharmacol *25*, 667–672 (1983)

(4) Decousus, H. A., Croze, M., Levi, F. A., Jaubert, J. G., Perpoint, B. M., DeBonadonna, J. F., Reinberg, A. and Queneau, P. M.: Circadian Changes in Anticoagulant Effect of Heparin Infused at a Constant Rate. Brit. Med. J. *290*, 341–344 (1985)

(5) Dethlefsen, U. and Repges, R.: Ein neues Therapieprinzip bei nächtlichem Asthma. Med. Klin. *80*, 44–47 (1985)

(6) English, J., Dunne, M., Marks, V.: Diurnal Variation in Prednisolone Kinetics. Clin. Pharmacol. Ther. 33, 381–385 (1983)

(7) Floyer, J.: A Treatise of the Asthma. Wilkin, London, 1698

(8) Haus, E., Nicolau, G. Y., Lakatua, D., Sakkett-Lundeen, L.: Reference Values for Chronopharmacology. Annual Review of Chronopharmacology *4*, 333–424 (1988)

(9) Hrushesky, W. J. M.: The Clinical Application of Chronobiology of Oncology. Am. J. Anat. *168*, 519–542 (1983)

(10) Hrushesky, W. J. M.: The Clinical Application of Chronobiology to Oncology. Am. J. Anat. *168*, 44–47 (1985)

(11) Kaukel, E., Koppermann, E. and Schrumm, C. H.: Zirkadiane Unterschiede in der Pharmakokinetik des Theophyllins. Atemw. Lungenkrh. *10*, 68–73 (1984)

(12) Lemmer, B. and Labrecque, G.: Chronopharmacology and Chronotherapeutics. Chronopharmacology International Vol. *4* No. 3, pp 319–329, 1987

(13) Lemmer, B.: The Chronopharmacology of Cardiovascular Medications. Ann. Rev. Chronopharmacol. *2*, 199–228 (1986)

(14) Markiewicz, A. and Semonowicz, K.: Time-Dependant Changes in the Pharmacokinetics of Aspirin. Int. J. Clin. Pharm. Biopharm. *17*, 409–411 (1979)

(15) Martin, R. J., Cicutto, L. C., Ballard, R. D., Szefler, S. J.: Airway Inflammation in Nocturnal Asthma. Am. Rev. Respir. Dis. *137*, 284 (1988)

(16) Mc Allister, W. A. C., Mitchell, D. M. and Collins, J. V.: Prednisolone Pharmacokinetics Compared Between Night and Day in Asthmatic and Normal Subjects. Br. J. Clin. Pharmacol. *11*. 303–304 (1981)

(17) Merki, H., Witzel, L., Harre, K., Scheurle, E., Bauerfeind, P., Blum, A. L. and Roehmel, J.: Circadian Pattern of Intragastric Acidity in Duodenal Ulcer (DU) Patients. A Comparison With Healthy Controls (HC). Gastroenterology *90*, 1549 (1986)

(18) Merki, H., Witzel, L., Harre, K., Scheurle, E., Bauerfeind, P., Blum, A. L. and Roehmel, J.: Single Dose Treatment With H_2-Receptor Antagonists. Is Bedtime Administration Too Late? Gastroenterology *90*, 1550 (1986)

(19) Mittler, M. M., Kripke, D. F.: Circadian Variation in Myocardial Infarction. N. Engl. J. Med. *314*, 1187–1188 (1986)

(20) Moore, J. G., Halberg, F.: Circadian Rhythm of Gastric Acid Secretion in Active Duodenal Ulcer: Chronobiological Statistical Characteristics and Comparison of Acid Secretory and Plasma Gastrin Patterns with Healthy Subjects and Post-Vagotomy and Pyloroplasty Patients. Chronobiology International *4*, 101–110 (1987)

(21) Morselli, P. L. and Marc, V.: Metabolism of Exogenous Cortisol in Humans – Diurnal Variations in Plasma Disappearance Rate. Biochem. Pharmacol. *19*, 1643–1647 (1970)

(22) Prevost, R. J., Smolensky, M. H., Reinberg, A., Raymer, W. J., Mc Govern, J. P.: Circadian Rhythm of Respiratory Distress in Asthmatic, Bronchitic, and Emphysematic Patients. In: Recent Advances in the Chronobiology of Allergy and Immunology Ed. by Smolensky, M. H., Reinberg, A., Mc Govern, J. P. Pergamon Press, Oxford, 1980, pp. 237–250

(23) Review: Smolensky, H. M., D'Alonzo, G. E., Kunkel, G. and Barnes, P. J.: Day – Night Patterns in Bronchial Patency and Dyspnoea: Basis for Once-Daily and Unequally Divided Twice-Daily Theophylline Dosing Schedules. Chronobiology International Vol. *4*, 303–317 (1987)

(24) Scott, P. H., Tabachnik, E., MacLeod, S., Correia, J., Newth, C. and Levison, H.: Sustained Release Theophylline for Childhood Asthma: Evidence for circadian variations of theophylline pharmacokinetics. J. Pediatr. *99*, 476–479 (1981)

(25) St-Pierre, M. V., Spino, M., Isles, A. F., Tesoro, A., MacLeod, S. M.: Temporal Variation in the Dispositon of Theophylline and its Metabolites. Clin. Pharmacol. Ther. *38*, 89–95 (1985)

(26) Uematsu, T., Follath, F., Vozeh, S.: Circadian Changes in the Absorption and Elimination of Theophylline in Patients with Bronchial Obstruction. Eur. J. Clin. Pharmacol. *30*. 309–312 (1986)

VI. Pharmacokinetic Characteristics of Controlled Release Products and Their Biostatistical Analysis

V. W. Steinijans, Konstanz

Summary

In order to assess and compare the controlled release of various formulations in vivo, suitable pharmacokinetic characteristics are needed. During the biopharmaceutical development of a controlled release product, single-dose studies are performed first. The pharmacokinetic profile of the final controlled release product and its dosage regimen should be compared under steady-state conditions with that of a conventional formulation or with another controlled release product. Apart from conventional characteristics such as AUC, t_{max} and C_{max}, alternative characteristics are considered such as residual concentration at the end of the dosage interval, peak-trough fluctuation in steady-state, plateau time, statistical moments, in-vivo input functions and intravenous infusion schemes which mimic the concentration/time profile after oral administration of the controlled release formulation. With regard to the experimental design and the biostatistical analysis of comparative studies, reference is made to the APV-Guideline on bioequivalence studies.

1. General Considerations

The objective of developing a controlled release product is prolongation of the drug's action and/or truncation of side effects which are caused by concentration peaks. Both aspects – better tolerability and reduced frequency of dosing – improve patient compliance (1, 13). Even if a so-called "therapeutic window" is not known explicitly, an implicit relation between effect and/or side effect and serum concentration is assumed. This paper does not deal with the complex relation between the time courses of serum concentrations and pharmacodynamic effects. It is confined to the pharmacokinetic characterization of controlled release products and their comparison, in particular with regard to bioavailability/bioequivalence studies.

During the biopharmaceutical development of a controlled release product, single-dose pharmacokinetic studies are usually performed; however, the final formulation should be compared under steady-state conditions with a conventional formulation and its dosage scheme or with another controlled release product serving as reference (7). Suitable pharmacokinetic characteristics are given for both, single- and multiple-dose studies. Besides characteristics of the intentionally modified rate of release also those of the extent of release are discussed, since the latter may also be affected by modifying the release rate.

Appropriate experimental designs and statistical evaluation techniques are given in accordance with existing guidelines, e. g. the APV-Guideline (6).

2. Pharmacokinetic characteristics of controlled release products

The pharmacokinetic characteristics under consideration should not only allow to assess the "strength" of the controlled release but should also enable the comparison between formulations with regard to rate and extent of absorption, i.e. bioavailability/bioequivalence. The characteristics can be considered as parameters which are derived from the concentration/time profiles; however, in this paper, the expression "parameter" is reserved for parameters of the statistical distribution of a characteristic.

Two types of characteristics have to be distinguished: those depending on specific pharmacokinetic compartment models and those depending on the weaker assumption of linear disposition kinetics (distribution and elimination). In this paper, the characteristics are presented separately for single- and multiple-dose studies.

3. Characteristics after single dose

The conventional characteristics of the pharmacokinetic profile after a single oral dose include AUC (area under the curve) as measure of the extent of absorption, and time, t_{max}, and height, C_{max}, of the maximum serum concentration as measures of the rate of absorption (Fig. 1). However, a reduction of C_{max} is not necessarily due to a reduced rate of absorption alone, but may also be due to a reduced extent of absorption. In the case of an adequate sampling scheme, t_{max} and C_{max} may be obtained directly from the measured concentrations.

The calculation of the total AUC from zero to infinity is usually performed as follows (6): AUC $(0, t_z)$, the area under the curve from zero to t_z, the time

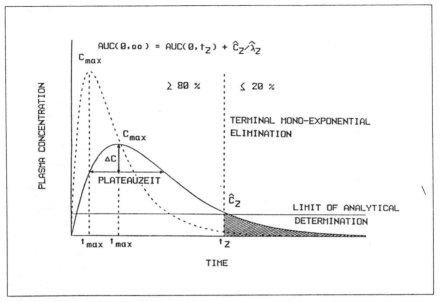

Fig. 1: Typical concentration/time profiles for a conventional (broken line) and an controlled release formulation (solid line). The time of the last measurement above the analytical limit of determination is denoted by t_z, the corresponding concentration by C_z, its estimation by the terminal log-linear regression by $\hat{C}_z$; ΔC denotes a clinically predetermined difference from the maximum concentration C_{max}. The plateau time is defined as the time span during which the concentration deviates from C_{max} by less than ΔC (From Pabst, J., ref. 12).

of the last measurement above the limit of analytical determination, is calculated by the linear trapezoidal rule. In the case of a terminal mono-exponential concentration/time course, the extrapolation to infinity, i.e. $AUC\,(t_z, \infty)$, is calculated by means of $\hat{C}_z/\hat{\lambda}_z$, where $\hat{\lambda}_z$ denotes the terminal rate constant estimated by logarithmic linear regression, and $\hat{C}_z$ denotes the concentration estimated at t_z by means of this regression line. In order to avoid any bias, $\hat{C}_z$ instead of C_z is also used in the determination of $AUC\,(O, t_z)$. The total AUC is then calculated as follows:

$$AUC = AUC\,(O, oo)$$
$$= AUC\,(O, t_z) + AUC\,(t_z, \infty)$$
$$= AUC\,(O, t_z) + \hat{C}_z/\hat{\lambda}_z.$$

The $AUC\,(O, t_z)$ obtained from the measured concentrations should account for at least 80% of the total AUC (6). Only if the pharmacokinetic model is definitely known, the AUC may be calculated by means of model parameters.

This applies also to the absorption rate constant, k_{abs}, which assumes a first-order absorption. An additional difficulty appears if absorption rather than elimination becomes the rate limiting step and if this is reflected in the apparent elimination rate constant λ_z and not any more in k_{abs} (so-called flip-flop phenomenon). Therefore, $t_{1/2} = \ln 2/\hat{\lambda}_z$ is also called "apparent half-life of elimination".

Controlled release products are primarily developed in the case of an unfavourable ratio between elimination half-life and envisaged dosage interval. After a single administration, the residual concentration at the end of the intended dosage interval is a simple criterion to differentiate between various developments. If the residual concentration is expressed as percentage of the maximum concentration, it provides an indicator of the peak-trough fluctuation to be expected after multiple dosing.

Data on t_{max}, and summarizing statistics in particular, are only meaningful if the maximum concentration, C_{max}, is prominent and sufficiently documented by measurements in the vicinity of C_{max}. In the case of flat and possibly multiple maxima, which frequently occur with controlled release products, the plateau time is a more suitable characteristic than t_{max}. The plateau time is defined as the time span of one dosing cycle, e.g. within 24 hours, during which the serum concentration deviates from the maximum concentration by less than a clinically specified difference or percentage. In the case of a 50 per cent deviation from the maximum, the plateau time corresponds to the half-value duration (HVD) introduced by Meier et al. 1974 (11); Fig. 2.

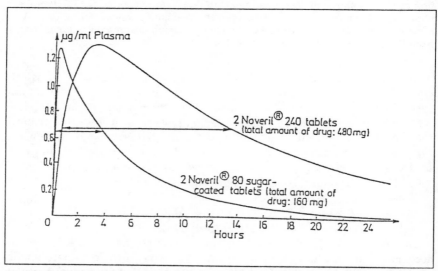

Fig. 2: Plasma concentrations of dibenzepin hydrochloride in man simulated on the basis of the mean values of pharmacokinetic characteristics for a conventional and an controlled release formulation (From Meier, J. et al., 11).

Meier and coworkers assumed that the conventional, i.e. non-controlled release product is effective in the neighbourhood of the maximum concentration. The time during which the plasma concentration is at least half of the effective maximum concentration was considered as pharmacokinetic correlate to the "width" of the efficacy range.

To assess the "strength" of the retardation, i.e. the controlled release, the above authors suggested the following procedure: The doses of the conventional and the controlled release product have to be chosen such that the maximum concentrations do not differ by more than 20%. Based on the ratio of the half-value durations,

R_{HVD} = HVD (controlled release product)/
$$\text{HVD (conventional dosage form)},$$

the following rating has been suggested:

$$\begin{aligned}
R_{HVD} &\leq 1 &&\text{no retardation} \\
R_{HVD} &= 1.5 &&\text{weak retardation} \\
R_{HVD} &= 2 &&\text{medium retardation} \\
R_{HVD} &\geq 3 &&\text{strong retardation.}
\end{aligned}$$

The half-value duration is only a special case of the more general concept of the plateau time. In the case of theophylline, for example, Jonkman and coworkers (5) originally considered the time interval during which the concentration exceeded 80% of the maximum concentration. Meanwhile, the value of 75% of the maximum concentration is widely accepted and the corresponding plateau time is denoted by $T75\%C_{max}$ (18).

Further characteristics of the pharmacokinetic profile after a single dose are the so-called statistical moments (14, 24) and characteristics derived therefrom such as the mean residence time (MRT) and the mean absorption time (MAT). If C(t) denotes the plasma concentration at time t and if integration extends from zero to infinity, then the following definitions hold (14):

area under the curve: $\quad\quad\quad$ $AUC = \int C(t)\, dt$
area under the moment curve: $\quad$ $AUMC = \int t\, C(t)\, dt$
mean residence time: $\quad\quad\quad$ $MRT = AUMC/AUC$
mean absorption time: $\quad\quad\quad$ $MAT = MRT_{p.o.} - (MRT_{i.v.} - MRT_{infusion\ device})$
$\quad\quad\quad\quad\quad\quad\quad\quad\quad\quad\quad\quad = MRT_{p.o.} - MRT_{i.v.\ adjusted}$

The mean residence time can also be considered as the expected value (first moment) of the distribution of the residence times of the molecules administered with one dose. In this case, the AUC-adjusted concentration/time curve serves as density function of the residence times (3).

With regard to the calculation of AUMC, a terminal mono-exponential concentration/time course with rate constand λ_z is usually assumed, firstly to ensure the existence of the corresponding integral, secondly to make the numerical calculation feasible. As before, let $\hat{\lambda}_z$ denote the least-squares estimation of λ_z and let $\hat{C}_z$ denote the estimated concentration at time t_z:

$\hat{C}_z = \hat{C}(t_z)$. Besides the combination of trapezoidal rule and subsequent extrapolation to infinity suggested by Riegelman and Collier (14), the method of the "area between the curves (ABC)" and the equivalent method of the "prospective area under the curve (PAUC)" suggested by Brockmeier (3) has proved useful in practice. If ABC (O, t) denotes the area between the polygon of the cumulative AUC up to time t, AUC(O, t), and the AUC extrapolated to infinity, AUC = AUC(O,oo), then the calculation of AUMC and ABC, respectively, is a follows (see also Fig. 3):

$$
\begin{aligned}
\text{AUMC} &= \text{AUMC (O, oo)} \\
&= \text{AUMC (O, } t_z) + t_z \, \hat{C}_z/\hat{\lambda}_z + \hat{C}_z/\hat{\lambda}_z^2 \\
&= \text{①} + \text{②} + \text{③} \\
&= \text{ABC (O, } t_z) + \hat{C}_z/\hat{\lambda}_z^2 \\
&= \text{ABC (O, oo)} \\
&= \text{ABC}
\end{aligned}
$$

The above formulae show that an unbiased estimation of the terminal rate constant is of utmost importance, since this estimate appears both in the numerator and the denominator of MRT, moreover not only linearly but also quadratically. When attempting the calculation of even higher moments (24) such as the variance of the residence time (VRT), which involve higher powers of λ_z, one should be aware of the underlying assumptions and possible numerical inaccuracies.

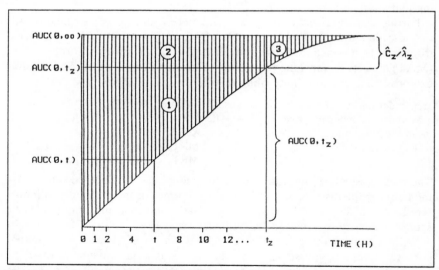

Fig. 3: Schematic representation of the calculation of ABC ("area between the curves" AUC(0,t) and AUC = AUC(0,oo)), which in turn is needed for the calculation of the mean residence time (MRT): MRT = ABC/AUC.

Despite its potential usefulness, the mean residence time has not yet gained widespread acceptance; apart from the numerical problems this may be due to the fact that summary tables of the mean residence times of widely used drugs and extended release formulations thereof are not available to date.

In contrast to the statistical moments, the in-vivo input functions have gained considerable importance for the characterization of controlled release products. Apart from the classical mass-balance methods according to Wagner-Nelsen ((22); one compartment body model) and Loo-Riegelman ((9); two-compartment body model), so-called numerical deconvolution methods (8), are used. The latter do not assume a specific compartmental model but merely linearity and time invariance of the disposition kinetics; for a review see the paper by Tucker (20), where the assumptions and the range of validity of the various procedures are given. All three methods require the knowledge of the disposition kinetics (distribution and elimination) which is usually derived from a reference experiment with intravenous administration.

The mass balance methods are based on the additivity of the amounts of drug which are still at the site of absorption, which are in the central compartment (including the sampling compartment) and, if necessary, in the peripheral compartment (not being available for measurements), and which have been excreted already.

The methods of deconvolution reconstruct the so-called "input-function" from the "response function", i.e. the concentration/time curve after oral administration, and the "weighting function", i.e. the concentration/time curve after intravenous administration (8). The input function can be considered as cumulative distribution function of intravenous boli, the superposition of which results in the concentration/time curve after oral administration. The calculation of the response function from the input- and weighting function is mathematically denoted as convolution, the recovery of the input function from the response- and weighting function as deconvolution (8).

Fig. 4, upper panel shows the concentration/time curves after oral administration of 30 mg urapidil as controlled release product and 10 mg urapidil as intravenous bolus injection in the same subject (25); the lower panel shows the in-vivo absorption profile calculated by means of the point-area method (21). Urapidil has a first-pass effect of 20–25% (25).

As the numerical deconvolution methods calculate the absorption rate in the n-th time interval on the basis of approximations in preceding time intervals, the choice of appropriate times of measurements is extremely important. Errors in the determination of the first value are carried over to all subsequent values. In view of this problem, numerical smoothing is frequently applied prior to deconvolution; in this way, a lot of interpolated values are added to sometimes only a few measured values. Therefore, the smoothing procedure used should at least be mentioned when presenting corresponding results;

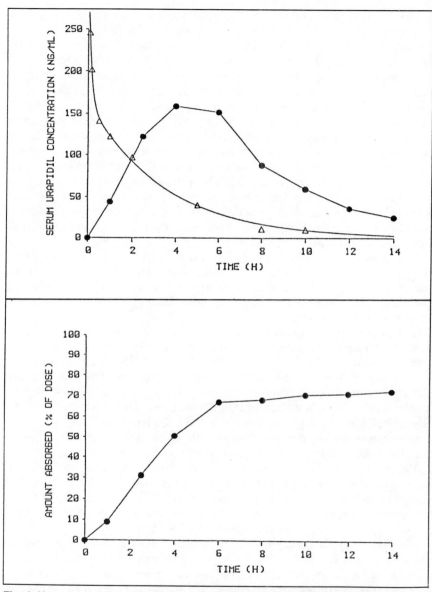

Fig. 4: Upper panel: Urapidil serum concentration following oral administration of 30 mg urapidil as controlled release capsule (●) and 10 mg urapidil as intravenous bolus injection (△). Lower panel: In-vivo input function (amount absorbed as per cent of the dose) calculated by means of numerical deconvolution (point-area method).

however, the correct solution of the problem is an appropriate sampling design, particularly in the absorption phase.

Langenbucher (8) suggested to apply the deconvolution method to obtain the in-vivo release profile of a controlled release product by comparing it with an orally administered solution. In dosing so, it is implicitly assumed that the conditions for absorption are the same in both cases. In this, however, is not the case, if the solution is primarily absorbed in the upper part of the small intestine, and if a major fraction of drug delivered by the controlled release product is absorbed in the large intestine. In this case, the in-vivo input function represents the rate limiting in-vitro release in the beginning, later on possibly the rate limiting absorption from the large intestine.

Another way to characterize a controlled release product after a single dose is the approximation of its concentration/time profile by that of an intravenous infusion scheme. In order to do so, the pharmacokinetics of the drug must be well known, both after intravenous administration and oral administration of the controlled release product. This sophisticated procedure, which is the experimental imitation of the theoretical concept of deconvolution, has the advantage that its results are easily understood, also by clinicians. For exam-

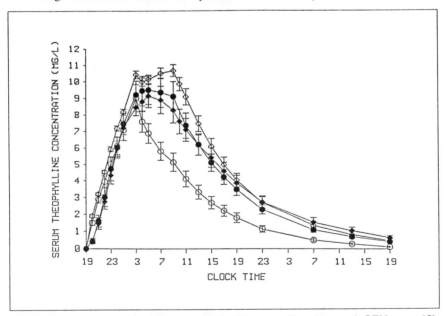

Fig. 5: Serum theophylline concentration/time profiles (mean ± SEM, n = 12) following oral administration of 750 mg theophylline as controlled release pellet formulation (● = Study 1, ◆ = Study 2), and intravenous infusion of 506 mg theophylline over 8 hours (○ = Study 1) and 749 mg over 14 hours with a reduced infusion rate after 8 hours (◇ = Study 2) (From Steinijans, V. W. et al., 19).

ple, the pharmacokinetic profile of a new controlled release theophylline pellet formulation could be approximated with sufficient accuracy by the following two-step infusion (Fig. 5): continuous infusion of approximately 70% of the dose over 8 hours, and continuous infusion of the remaining fraction of the dose over an additional 6 hours. Drug release by this infusion scheme can also be regarded as an infusion over 14 hours with a reduction of the infusion rate from 69 mg/h to 33 mg/h after 8 hours (19). This characterization of the controlled release product provides a deeper insight than the mere figure of a mean absorption time of 8 hours.

4. Characteristics after multiple dose

After multiple dosing of a controlled release product, the extent of absorption can be characterized by the AUC over one dosage interval τ or equivalently by the average concentration, $C_{av} = AUC/\tau$.

The conventional characteristics t_{max} and C_{max} are of limited value in the case of flat and sometimes multiple maxima. In this case, the plateau time is

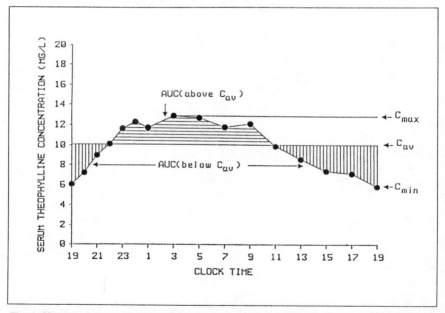

Fig. 6: Maximum, average and minimum serum concentrations during a 24-hour dose interval in steady state and areas above and below the average concentration, using a controlled release theophylline pellet formulation for once-daily dosing in the evening as an example.

particularly suited to characterize the "strength" of the controlled release; this can also be done by expressing the residual concentration at the end of the dosage interval in per cent of either the maximum or the average concentration. The rate of absorption, which ideally is release limited, can be expressed by the various peak-trough characteristics (18):

per cent peak-trough fluctuation:
$\%PTF = 100 \ (C_{max}-C_{min})/C_{av}$
per cent swing:
$\%swing = 100 \ (C_{max}-C_{min})/C_{min}$
per cent AUC-fluctuation:
$\%AUCF = 100 \ (AUC[above \ C_{av}] + AUC[below \ C_{av}])/AUC.$

Whereas the per cent peak-trough fluctuation and particularly the per cent swing are very sensitive to single measurements and their potential errors – C_{min} in particular –, the per cent AUC-fluctuation around C_{av} is a robust measure of the fluctuation of the serum concentrations ((2), (18); Fig. 6).

The various pharmacokinetic characteristics after single and multiple dose have been summarized in Tab. 1.

Tab. 1: Pharmacokinetic characteristics to assess controlled-release formulations

	Single-dose studies	Multiple-dose studies (steady state)
Conventional characteristics	AUC, t_{max}, C_{max} k_{abs}, λ_z and $t_{1/2}$	AUC or C_{av}, t_{max}, C_{max} k_{abs}, λ_z and $t_{1/2}$
Alternative characteristics	Residual concentration at the end of the proposed dosage interval in % of C_{max}	Residual concentration at the end of the dosage interval in % of C_{max} or C_{av}
	Plateau time (half-value duration, $T75\%C_{max}$)	Peak-trough characteristics (%peak-trough fluctuation, %swing, %AUC-fluctuation)
	Mean residence time (MRT) Mean absorption time (MAT)	Plateau time (Half-value duration, $T75\%C_{max}$)
	In-vivo inputfunction (Wagner-Nelson method, Loo-Riegelman method, Deconvolution)	
	Approximation of the serum concentration/time profile after p. o. administration by an i. v. infusion scheme	

5. Experimental designs for comparative studies of controlled release products

The same principles of experimental design which apply to comparative bioavailability/bioequivalence studies also apply to the comparison of controlled release products. They have been laid down in various guidelines, most precisely in the APV-Guideline (6) from which the following excerpt has been taken.

Due to marked inter-individual differences in absorption, distribution, metabolism and elimination of a drug, the crossover design is usually regarded as the appropriate one. If more than one test formulation is compared with the reference formulation, a multiple crossover design corresponding to the number of investigated formulations has to be chosen. The allocation of the subjects to the treatment sequences should be randomized. In the case of single-dose studies, the experimental periods have to be seperated by sufficiently long washout periods (of approximately 5 half-lives of elimination). In the case of multiple-dose pharmacokinetic studies in which investigations are performed only in steady state, which is reached after about 5 half-lives, a washout phase can be omitted.

In special cases, e.g. drugs with extremely slow elimination, a parallel group design may be indicated. The external experimental conditions (e.g. diet, fluid intake, physical activity) should be standardized between groups. The allocation of the subjects to the treatment groups should be randomized.

If linear pharmacokinetics (i.e. constant clearance) cannot be assumed, equal doses and dosage intervals must be chosen if similar pharmacokinetics profiles can be expected; otherwise, the dosage scheme has to be chosen such that the concentration/time profiles match each other as close as possible (cf. i.v. infusion scheme).

In the planning of a bioequivalence study, a sample size consideration should be performed. The number of subjects should be large enough to obtain sufficiently small probabilities of a decision for bioequivalence if it is actually not true and against bioequivalence if it is actually true. The number of subjects depends on the experimental design and a corresponding, a priori selected, statistical method of evaluation of the primary characteristic. If the evaluation is based on a linear model with normally distributed errors, the sample size depends directly on the unknown true difference between the two formulations and the true coefficient of variation. If bioequivalence is assessed by a sufficiently large Bayesian posterior probability, the nomograms provided by Fluehler et al. (4) may be used for sample size calculation. The reliability of the calculation should be checked by repeating it with the actual values obtained in the trial.

6. Evaluation procedures for comparative studies of controlled release products

With regard to the statistical evaluation, too, the principles of bioavailability/bioequivalence studies as laid down in the APV-Guideline (6) are applicable.

For the presentation of the results it is recommended to give the following values for each subject: sex, age, weight, height and relevant findings of the clinical examination. Apart from the treatment sequence and the individual concentration/time data and excretion data, the individual values of each characteristic should be given for each treatment period. Moreover, it is recommended to give the individual ratios test/reference for all characteristics, except for the discrete variable t_{max} which is best described by a frequency table. As a general principle it is recommended to determine the characteristic for each subject first, and then to perform the statistical analysis with the individual values.

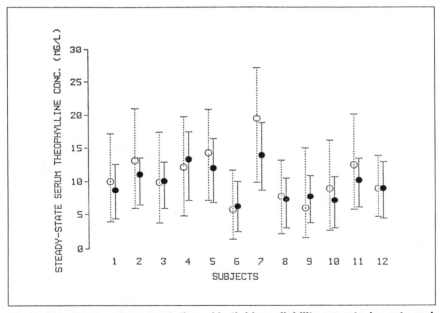

Fig. 7: Simultaneous representation of both bioavailability aspects, i.e. rate and extent of absorption, in the case of multiple-dose studies. For each of the 12 subjects participating in a randomized crossover study with two treatment periods of 7 days each (800 mg theophylline/day; ○ = reference formulation, ● = test formulation), the following characteristics are given: Maximum (peak), C_{max}, minimum (trough), C_{min}, and 24-hour time averaged concentration, C_{av}. C_{av} reflects the extent of absorption, the peak-trough difference $C_{max} - C_{min}$ the rate of absorption.

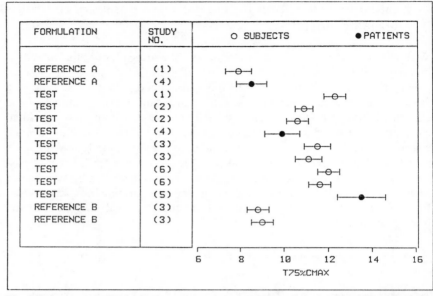

Fig. 8: Plateau time, T 75 % C$_{max}$, for various controlled release theophylline formulations after repeated once-daily evening administration. Results with identical study number refer to randomized crossover studies, in the case of the same formulation to two 24-hour steady-state profiles (○ = healthy subjects, ● = COPD patients).

As a descriptive summary of the pharmacokinetic results of a comparative study of two controlled release products under steady-state conditions, the simultaneous presentation of both bioavailability aspects, rate and extent of absorption, is particularly informative ((18); Fig. 7).

For a particular characteristic, a descriptive summary of various studies can be presented as in Fig. 8 (18). In the case of identical study designs, e. g. measurements every two hours during one steady-state dosage interval, this presentation provides a very simple descriptive metaanalysis.

With regard to the inference statistical analysis of comparative studies of controlled release products the same procedures as with bioequivalence studies can be used. The objective of a bioequivalence study is to show that with a sufficiently high probability the observed difference is within the bioequivalence range. To this end, a statistical test with the null-hypothesis "no difference between the formulations" is not suited.

A widely accepted decision rule leads to the acceptance of "bioequivalence", if either the symmetrical 95%-confidence interval or the shortest 90%-confidence interval for the ratio of the expected values of the primary characteristic is entirely in the bioequivalence range (10, 15, 16, 23).

Equivalent to the decision based on symmetrical 95%-confidence limits is the calculation of a Bayesian posterior probability of the least 0.95 that the true ratio lies within the bioequivalence range.

In order to control the probability of a decision for bioequivalence if it actually does not hold true, the following hypotheses haved to be considered: **Null hypothesis:** The ratio of the expected values of test and reference, μ_T/μ_R, exceeds the acceptable limits with regard to bioequivalence, $\theta_1 < \theta_2$:

$$H_o:\ \mu_T/\mu_R \leq \theta_1 \text{ or } \mu_T/\mu_R \geq \theta_2.$$

Alternative hypothesis: The ratio lies within the specified bioequivalance range:

$$\theta_1 < \mu_T/\mu_R < \theta_2.$$

The rejection of the null hypothesis implies bioequivalence, provided the type I error is controlled accordingly. In a recent paper by Schuirmann (15) the following procedure has been suggested: Two one-sided t-tests at level α (e. g. $\alpha = 0.05$) with the following null hypotheses are performed: H_{o1}: $\mu_T/\mu_R \leq \theta_1$, i. e. the ratio of the expected values of test and reference is smaller or equal to the lower bound θ_1; H_{o2}: $\mu_T/\mu_R \geq \theta_2$, i. e. the ratio is larger or equal to the upper bound θ_2. The rejection of both null hypotheses implies the decision for bioequivalence. Schuirmann has shown that with this procedure the probability of erroneously accepting bioequivalence is less or equal to α; moreover, this procedure is equivalent to the construction of a 1–2 α confidence interval which is entirely in the bioequivalance range. According to this, the conventional 1-α confidence intervals are conservative insofar as the probability of erroneously accepting bioequivalence is less or equal to $\alpha/2$. In the case of Westlake's shortest symmetrical 1-α confidence intervals this probability ranges between $\alpha/2$ and α.

7. Discussion and Conclusions

An overview of conventional and alternative pharmacokinetic characteristics of controlled release products is given. The presentation focusses after single dosing on the ideally release-limited absorption and after multiple dosing on the peak-trough characteristics. In both cases, the "strength" of the controlled release may be characterized by the plateau time and the residual concentration at the end of the dosage interval.

The mathematical algorithms to calculate the various characteristics are presented either directly or by referring to relevant literature. The theoretical assumptions as well as further conditions frequently assumed in practice are described. The importance of appropriate experimental design and statistical analysis is emphasized.

The assessment of the various procedures shows which characteristics are particularly suitable for such different aspects as, for example, strength of controlled release, completeness of absorption and fluctuation of serum concentrations during the intended dosage interval. The biopharmaceutical development of a controlled release product has to be considered as a balanced optimization of such partial aspects, the weighting of which should be based on clinical-pharmacological requirements.

8. Literature

(1) Ayd, F. J.: Single daily dose of antidepressants (editorial). JAMA *230*, 263–264 (1974)
(2) Boxenbaum, H.: Pharmacokinetic determinants in the design and evaluation of sustained-release dosage forms. Pharm. Res. *2*, 82–88 (1984)
(3) Brockmeier, D.: Die Bedeutung statistischer Momente der Verweildauer für die Pharmakokinetik und Biopharmazie. Inaugural Dissertation, Fachbereich Humanmedizin, Justus-Liebig-Universität Gießen, 1982
(4) Fluehler, H., Grieve, A. P., Mandallaz, D., Mau, J., Moser, H. A.: Bayesian approach to bioequivalance assessment: an example. J. Pharm. Sci. *72*, 1178–1181 (1983)
(5) Jonkman, J. H. G., Berg, W. C., Grimberg, N., de Vries, K., de Zeeuw, R. A., Schoenmaker, R.: Disposition and clinical pharmacokinetics of theophylline after administration of a new sustained release tablet. Eur. J. Clin. Pharmacol. *21*, 39–44 (1981)
(6) Junginger, H.: Studies on bioavailability and bioequivalence. APV guideline. Drugs Made in Germany *30*, 161–166 (1987)
(7) Koch-Weser, J., Schechter, P. J.: Slow-release preparations in clinical perspective. pp. 217–227 in Drug Absorption (Eds. Prescott, L. F., Nimmo, W. S.), Adis Press, New York, 1979
(8) Langenbucher, F.: Numerical convolution/deconvolution as a tool for correlating in vitro with in vivo drug availability. Pharm. Ind. *44*, 1166–1172 (1982)
(9) Loo, J. C. K., Riegelman, S.: New method for calculating the intrinsic absorption rate of drugs. J. Pharm. Sci. *57*, 918–928 (1968)
(10) Mandallaz, D., Mau, J.: Comparison of different methods for decision-making in bioequivalence assessment. Biometrics *37*, 213–222 (1981)
(11) Meier, J., Nüesch, E., Schmidt, R.: Pharmacokinetic criteria for the evaluation of

retard formulations. Eur. J. Clin. Pharmacol. *7*, 429–432 (1974)
(12) Pabst, J.: Pharmakokinetische Parameter zur Bioäquivalenzentscheidung unter Berücksichtigung von Arzneiformen mit modifizierter Freisetzung. Apotheken Report *30*, 20–27 (1986)
(13) Porter, A. M.: Drug defaulting in a general practise. Br. Med. J. *1*, 218–222 (1969)
(14) Riegelman, S., Collier, P.: The application of statistical moment theory to the evaluation of in vivo dissolution time and absorption time. J. Pharmacokinet. Biopharm. *8*, 509–534 (1980)
(15) Schuirmann, D. J.: A comparison of the two one-sided tests procedure and the power approach for assessing the equivalence of average bioavailability. J. Pharmacokinet. Biopharm. *15*, 657–680 (1987)
(16) Steinijans, V. W., Diletti, E.: Statistical analysis of bioavailability studies: parametric and nonparametric confidence intervals. Eur. J. Clin. Pharmacol. *24*, 127–136 (1983)
(17) Steinijans, V. W.: Verfahren zur statistischen Bewertung von Bioäquivalenzstudien. Apotheken Report *30*, 28–39 (1986)
(18) Steinijans, V. W., Trautmann, H., Johnson, E., Beier, W.: Theophylline steady-state pharmacokinetics: recent concepts and their application in chronotherapy of reactive airway diseases. Chronobiol. Int. *4*, 331–347 (1987a)
(19) Steinijans, V. W., Schulz, H.-U., Böhm, A., Beier, W.: Absolute bioavailability of theophylline from a sustained-release formulation using different intravenous reference infusions. Eur. J. Clin. Pharmacol. *33*, 523–526 (1987b)
(20) Tucker, G. T.: The determination of in vivo drug absorption rate. Acta Pharm. Technol. *29*, 159–164 (1983)
(21) Vaughan, D. P., Dennis, M.: Mathematical

basis of point-area deconvolution method for determining in vivo input functions. J. Pharm. Sci. *67*, 663–665 (1978)

(22) Wagner, J. G., Nelson, E.: Per cent absorbed time plots derived from blood level and/or urinary excretion data. J. Pharm. Sci. *52*, 610–611 (1963)

(23) Westlake, W. J.: Statistical aspects of comparative bioavailability trials. Biometrics *35*, 273–280 (1979)

(24) Yamaoka, K., Nakagawa, T., Uno, T.: Statistical moments in pharmacokinetics. J. Pharmacokinet. Biopharm. *6*, 547–558 (1978)

(25) Zech, K., Sturm, E., Steinijans, V. W.: Pharmakokinetik und Metabolismus von Urapidil (Ebrantil) bei Tier und Mensch. S. 50–64 in Urapidil, Darstellung einer neuen antihypertensiven Substanz (Eds. Kaufmann, W., Bruckschen, E. G.). Excerpta Medica Amsterdam, 1982

VII. The Significance of Nutrition for the Biopharmaceutical Characteristics of Oral Controlled Release Products and Enteric Coated Dosage Forms

I. E. Walter-Sack, Heidelberg

Summary

*The systemic availability of an active compound in the fasting state may differ from the plasma concentration time course in the fed state. **"Fasting" drug application** implies the stomach to be empty prior to dosing, and in addition it implies that the fasting gastric motility pattern is maintained after drug administration. Therefore drug intake with any kind of nutrient-containing material, for example beverages like fruit juice, cannot be considered as fasting application and consequently is not a valid reference procedure for evaluation of the effects of a meal. Ingestion of food stimulating gastric acid secretion like coffee or tea prior to drug administration also can influence gastric emptying. The **consequences of concurrent intake of food** vary with the pharmaceutical properties of a particular medicinal product and therefore have to be evaluated separately for each dosage form. In addition variations of the systemic availability depend on the composition of food, so that the effects documented in a certain study not necessarily are representative. Apart from drug absorption nutrition also can affect drug elimination; diet-induced variations of the elimination capacity are relevant irrespectively of the route of drug administration and can interfere with the assessment of the absolute as well as the relative systemic availability. General agreement should be intended on the standards required for assessing the systemic availability in order to generate reproducible and representative information. The diet provided during the actual sampling periods should meet the nutritional standards set for the majority of the western population (no more than 30% of energy derived from fat). The individual diet also should be in accordance with modern dietary recommendations and remain essentially unchanged during the entire duration of a biopharmaceutical study. The use of high fat meals should be abandoned, because it does not meet adequate standards. – Gastric motor function in the fasting state is fundamentally different from the fed state. This has major implications for gastric handling of **oral controlled*** *release and enteric coated products. Two principally different types of formulations have to be considered: Single unit and multiple unit forms. Controlled release preparations do allow the active constituent to become available in the systemic circulation during the digestive period. Coingestion of food can remain without effect, increase or reduce the rate and/or extent of systemic availability of the active ingredient. Data so far available do not indicate a typical pattern of food effects with single unit or multiple unit controlled release forms and therefore do not suggest a general advantage of either dosage form as far as the susceptability to an influence of food is concerned. In drugs characterized by a high so-called first pass metabolism the effects of a meal can be delivery rate dependent (rapid or slow release preparation), and in addition vary with the route of drug administration. Single unit enteric coated products constitute a different pharmaceutical entity in that the active ingredient cannot become available in the circulation during the digestive period. Various clinical problems may arise mainly from the use of single unit dosage forms; patients with gastric emptying disorders probably are at particular risk. Specification of the formulation is necessary and has to be included into the product information in order to allow selection of an individually safe dosage form.*

1. General considerations

The biopharmaceutical characteristics of drugs generally are assessed by determining the systemic availability, as opposed to the availability for absorption or the availability at the site of action. Several variables may be combined to define "bioavailability" (1, 2, 3, 21), even though they differ in their pharmacologic and therapeutic implications; confining the definition to the particular variable which actually is measured (the systemic availability) would provide a definition of bioavailability more readily applicable to practice (98).

The **systemic availability** – the rate and the extent to which an active constituent becomes available in the general circulation – represents the net effect of drug uptake into and drug elimination from the circulation (Fig. 1). Following oral application, drug influx is a function of the rate and the extent of absorption from the gastrointestinal tract and the presystemic degradation during the first passage of the gastrointestinal mucosa and the liver (and possibly the lung); drug efflux mainly is related to the capacity of the liver and the kidney to remove a substance from the systemic circulation. Each of these processes can be modified by nutrition (87, 88): Depending on the phar-

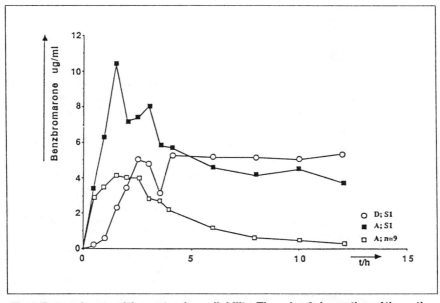

Fig. 1: Determinants of the systemic availability: The role of <u>absorption</u> of the active ingredient from various formulations is illustrated by comparison of curve A;S1 and D;S1 showing benzbromarone plasma concentrations in the same subject (S1) after fasting application of two different brands (A and D) both containing the same amount of drug; the <u>rate</u> of systemic availability was remarkably different: Maximum plasma concentrations were lower and the time to achieve peak concentrations was prolonged with D; in addition the increment of plasma concentrations per unit of time was less. The significance of drug <u>elimination</u> from the systemic circulation is illustrated by comparison of curves A;S1 and A;n=9: Plasma concentrations of benzbromarone following fasting application of brand A to the subject mentioned before, being a deficient metaboliser (A;S1) and to 9 individuals being extensive metabolisers (A;n=9) revealed an about 3-fold difference in the <u>extent</u> of systemic availability during the first 12 hours after dosing (From Walter-Sack, I. et al., ref. 87). Like in this case variations of drug elimination can be permanent, but also can arise temporarily from changes of nutrition (From Tranvouez, J. L. et al., ref. 85).

maceutical properties of oral preparations **concomitant food intake** can affect the availability of the active ingredient for absorption, and thereby either increase or decrease the rate and/or the extent of systemic availability as compared to fasting conditions. In addition concurrent ingestion of a meal can diminish the presystemic elimination of drugs characterized by a high so-called first pass metabolism, if conventional immediate release preparations are used (54, 55, 67, 86); the extent of reduction appears to be related to the protein content of the meal (86). Food intake has no effect when a controlled release preparation is applied (10, 46): The rate of release of the active constituent determines whether food alters drug elimination from the **portal** circulation or not. Diet-induced variations of drug clearance from the **systemic** circulation also may be a consequence of acute effects of a single meal, but in addition can be due to adherance to a particular dietary regimen. Acute effects of a meal have been described for instance for propranolol and gentamycin: The systemic clearance of propranolol is enhanced shortly after food ingestion, probably as a consequence of an intermittent rise of hepatic perfusion (67); renal excretion of gentamycin varies with glomerular filtration, possibly as a function of protein intake (19).

The impact of certain **dietary patterns** on drug elimination has been documented in healthy individuals as well as in patients: a reduction of energy intake below the individual needs and/or a diminished intake of protein results in a decreased capacity to metabolize antipyrine (8, 33, 40, 85); increasing the protein supply is associated with enhanced antipyrine clearance (unless there is a severe defect in certain malnourished patients). Theophylline biotransformation similarly changes with the protein content of the diet (33). Apart from nutrients some nonnutritive food components also can influence drug metabolism; for example a high intake of polycyclic hydrocarbons due to ingestion of charcoal-broiled food stimulates phenacetin degradation (15). In addition the renal excretion of certain drugs may be related to particular dietary patterns (88).

Deviations of the elimination capacity are relevant irrespectively of the route of drug administration; since they are important for oral as well as for parenteral dosage forms, dietary changes can interfere in several ways with the assessment of the relative and the absolute availability. Therefore nutrition needs to be well controlled during biopharmaceutical studies. This implies, that the diet is standardized during the actual sampling periods as well as during the drug-free intervals: The individual diet should essentially remain unchanged during the entire period of investigation, beginning about one week prior to drug application, and should provide adequate amounts of nutrients while avoiding undesirable dietary components (89). During the various sampling periods the composition of the meals should be constant, because the secretory and the motor responses of the upper gastrointestinal tract vary with the physico-chemical properties of food (47, 49, 58).

Gastric motor function is a major determinant of the availability of a drug for absorption, since the stomach controls the delivery of the active constituent to the site of absorption in the small intestine. Fasting gastric motility is fundamentally different from the motor activity of the stomach during the digestive period. **"Fasting" drug application** therefore not only implies the stomach to be empty prior to drug ingestion, but in addition implies that fasting motility is maintained **after** drug administration.

2. Gastric emptying of liquids and solids

The human stomach can be divided into two functional compartments – the proximal and the distal stomach. Emptying of liquids is related to the gastro-duodenal pressure gradient which is controlled by the proximal stomach, whereas emptying of solids is a function of the contractile activity of the distal stomach (30, 39, 47, 58, 63, 93, 95).

The gastroduodenal transport of **liquids** in the fasting state does not differ from the digestive period in so far as liquids can leave the stomach practically at any time – the rate of emptying being a function of the volume and the composition of the liquid phase of gastric contents, mainly the acidity, osmolarity, and nutrient density. Inert liquids which do not interrupt fasting motility, for instance water or isotonic saline (73), are delivered to the duodenum quite rapidly (9, 47, 58, 81); the kinetics of this process can be best described by a **monoexponential** function (14, 25, 81). Liquids which contain nutrients – carbohydrates, fat, or protein – inhibit the typical fasting motor activity of the stomach and are retained for longer periods of time (20, 73). An emulsion of fat and water is emptied more slowly than water alone, but more rapidly than fat alone (47). With homogeneous meals the liquid and the solid phase can leave the stomach together (16), whereas liquids are emptied separately from solid food, when ingested as part of an ordinary solid-liquid meal (17); however in this case the type of solid food influences the rate of removal of liquids (23).

Gastric emptying of **solids** in the fasting state is fundamentally different from the fed state, in that the **pattern** of gastroduodenal transport differs: **Fasting** motor activity is characterized by typical electromechanical cycles; one cycle is divided into 4 phases: During phase 1 and 2 only little electrical activity is observed, which is not associated with muscular contraction waves. Only during phase 3 a high electrical activity arises, which is accompanied by propulsive peristaltic waves capable to transport solid material from the stomach into the duodenum. This may be followed by a short phase 4 just prior to recurrence of the next cycle. The duration of an entire cycle on average is 2 hours (varying from 1 to 3 hours), whereas phase 3 is no longer than about 5 to 15 minutes (47, 58, 63, 73, 93). Since propulsive contraction waves only are induced during phase 3, solid material in the fasting state will only be emptied from the stomach about every 2 hours. Consequently gastric residence time of solid material during the fasting period depends on the time interval between ingestion and the recurrence of a phase 3 contraction, and so by chance may vary between a few minutes and 2 (–3) hours.

The motor activity of the distal stomach during fasting is confined to the transport function; in contrast the **digestive** motility is characterized by a continuous mixing, grinding, and sieving action, thereby altering the structure of solid material prior to the delivery to the small intestine. This motor action results in a brake down of solids to a particle size of 1–2 mm (30, 47, 58, 63,

93, 95). Only solids which are "liquefied" in this way can leave the stomach **during** the digestive period; larger particles are retained for further degradation. Solids which cannot at all be reduced to the particle size required for emptying during the digestive period – which are "indigestible" in this sense – cannot leave the stomach as long as digestion still goes on. Consequently nondegradable solids remain in the stomach until fasting motility recurs, then being removed by the first phase 3 contraction wave. This has important implications for single unit drug dosage forms.

Delivery of the liquefied components of gastric contents to the duodenum occurs about **linearly** with time, the rate of transport being related to several factors: Acidity, osmolarity, nutrient density, and the structure of solid food – the digestibility – are important determinants of gastric emptying (9, 14, 25, 30, 47, 58, 63, 75, 93). With increasing energy density of gastric contents the volume delivered to the duodenum per unit of time decreases; isoenergetic solutions of fat, carbohydrates, and protein (for instance 36 Kcal/dl, equivalent to 4 g fat/dl, 9 g carbohydrate/dl, or 9 g protein/dl) leave the stomach at similar rates (31, 58). This also applies to mixtures of nutrients: for example the average time required to empty a meal equivalent to 345–395 Kcal was observed to be 139–140 minutes independently of the composition of food: There was no difference between a no-fat meal and a high-fat meal (38). With a test meal equivalent to 560 Kcal a mean duration of the digestive period of 160–209 minutes was found (48).

When the ingested solid food pieces are large, more time is required for adequate reduction of particle size and delivery of the material to the duodenum than with initially small particles – the digestive period is prolonged (28); by homogenizing a solid-liquid meal, gastric emptying is speeded up, gastric residence time is shortened (49). Since the physical properties of solid food determine the time necessary for brake down, the structure of the raw product (for instance the content of dietary fiber), the way of food preparation, and the individual extent of chewing can modify the duration of the fed state. Intake of additional meals prior to completion of the digestive process maintains the digestive motility pattern (extends the digestive period), and thereby delays removal of nondegradable solids irrespectively of particle size, if it exceeds 2 mm (80); frequent feeding (every 2–3 h) can prolong the digestive period beyond 14.5 h (60).

In healthy individuals the stomach acts as a reservoir for food, adapting the delivery of nutrients and fluid to the absorptive capacity of the small intestine. When nutrients are present in the jejunum or ileum (when absorption is incomplete), gastric emptying is inhibited (27, 57, 71). This mechanism is likely to explain why the "head" of a meal appears to have a shorter transit time through the stomach and the small intestine than the remainder of a meal (71). Furthermore nutrients in the ileum can delay gastric emptying of the subsequent meal (72).

3. Gastric handling of drugs

An active compound practically never can be administered on its own, but has to be imbedded or dissolved in excipients. The rate and the extent of systemic availability of the active ingredient therefore are more characteristic of a pharmaceutical formulation than of a substance. Primarily the type of excipients and the manufacturing procedures determine the release kinetics of a dosage form; however these can be modified by nutrition, for instance when oral preparations and food are ingested concurrently. Food can affect the systemic availability of a drug by a change of the availability for absorption, either as a consequence of an alteration of the intragastric release of the active ingredient, its dissolution or stability, or the time course of the gastroduodenal transport (87). Furthermore the systemic availability may vary due to an influence of a meal on presystemic drug elimination (88).

3.1 When oral immediate release preparations are administered **fasting** with an adequate volume of water, an aqueous solution will be formed quickly within the stomach. This type of inert solutions can leave the stomach very fast, as shown by marker drugs like paracetamol: The half life of absorption of paracetamol in the small intestine is 6–7 minutes (13); since the transmucosal

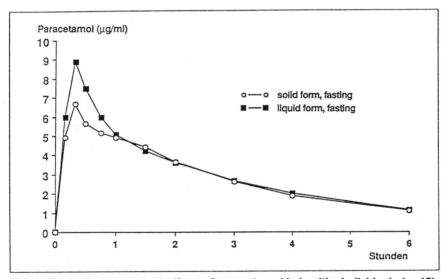

Fig. 2: Mean plasma concentrations of paracetamol in healthy individuals (n=12) following fasting administration of a liquid and a solid immediale release preparation together with 200 ml of water; the rate of systemic availability was similar with the two dosage forms: peak concentrations were achieved within 20 minutes after dosing (From Walter-Sack, I., ref. 88).

transport is so rapid, the systemic availability of paracetamol reflects the sum of events prior to the actual absorption process – the intragastric formation of a paracetamol solution plus the gastroduodenal transport of the dissolved drug. When a liquid or a solid rapid release preparation of paracetamol was given fasting with 200 ml of water, maximum plasma concentrations were achieved within 20–35 minutes after dosing ([91], Fig. 2). When the availability of an active compound for absorption is less, either as a consequence of the physico-chemical properties of the substance or differences of the pharmaceutical characteristics of various formulations, for instance of benzbromarone, more time is required to achieve peak concentrations ([90], Fig. 1).

Ingestion of food alters the intragastric environment for the release and dissolution of the active ingredient, and in addition induces the digestive pattern of gastric emptying; this can result in an alteration of the systemic availability as compared to fasting drug application: When a liquid preparation of paracetamol was administered with a low fiber formula diet, the rate of systemic availability was decreased: Maximal paracetamol plasma concentra-

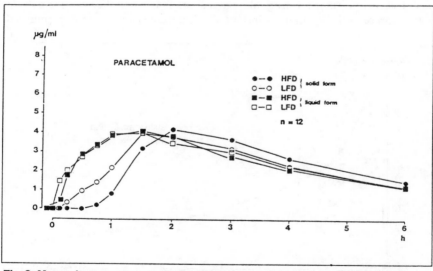

Fig. 3: Mean plasma concentrations of paracetamol in healthy subjects (n=12) following application of a liquid and a solid rapid release preparation; instead of water 200 ml of either a low fiber formula diet (LFD, Fresubin®) or a formula diet enriched in insoluble fiber (HFD, Fresubin plus®) were coingested. Both diets equally reduced the rate of systemic availability as compared to fasting application, if the liquid dosage form of paracetamol was used; but there was a differential effect of the two diets, when the solid paracetamol preparations was substituted for the liquid form (From Walter-Sack, I., ref. 89).

tions were lower than after fasting drug intake, and the time span necessary to achieve peak concentrations was prolonged to about 1.5 hours; with a formula diet enriched in small particles of dietary fiber an equivalent plasma concentration time course of paracetamol was observed ([92], Fig. 3). Apart from the content of dietary fiber the two test meals differed in the pattern of fatty acids, amino acids, and sugars, but were identical in the total amount of carbohydrates, fat, and protein (constant nutrient relations), total volume (200 ml), energy density, and osmolarity. The differences of meal composition obviously did not result in differences of drug delivery to the duodenum as long as a **liquid** preparation of paracetamol was used. However when a **solid** dosage form was substituted for the liquid preparation, the systemic availability of paracetamol was affected in a differential way: Following coadministration of the immediate release tablet and the low fiber diet, drug absorption was retarded to a greater extent than with the liquid paracetamol preparation; during the first 20 minutes after dosing paracetamol only was detectable in traces (Fig. 3). With the high fiber diet a further delay was observed; the drug did not appear in the systemic circulation for about 45 minutes following application, and time to reach maximal concentrations was extended to 2.5 hours. The data illustrate, that **the response of the systemic availability to concurrent food intake varies with the composition of the meal, but in addition is a function of the pharmaceutical formulation.** This implies, that the "food effects" documented a certain study reflect the interaction of a particular drug product and a particular test meal, which not necessarily is representative for other pharmaceutical formulations or for test meals of different composition.

3.2 With oral controlled release products two fundamentally different formulation principles have to be considered: **Single unit** forms and **multiple unit** forms (3). The difference of the pharmaceutical formulation has major implications for the mechanism of gastric emptying of the solid matrix as well as the active ingredient.

Single unit controlled release products do not decompose into smaller particles, but will release the active compound within the stomach. Gastric emptying is very rapid for inert aqueous solutions; therefore the release of the active ingredient after fasting application is likely to be the rate-limiting step for drug absorption. This may be different when the stomach contains liquid or solid food. Since the total amount of drug available for absorption is a function of time, gastric retention of single unit preparations can be crucial for the extent of systemic availability. Gastric residence time (GRT) of nondegradable dosage forms is related to the time interval between ingestion and recurrence of a gastric phase 3 contraction wave **irrespectively** of whether the product is administered fasting or during the digestive period; it can be estimated indirectly from data obtained with the Heidelberg capsule, a pH-sensitive radiotelemetric device considered to be representative for indigestible solids:

After fasting ingestion GRT of the capsule on average was 0.5 h; by a 285 kcal and a 500 kcal meal it was extended to 2.6 and 4.8 h respectively. Frequent feeding (every 2–3 h) resulted in prolongation of the mean GRT to more than 14.5 h (60). However there is an appreciable variation even following fasting application: Gastric retention of a placebo tablet (nondegradable matrix) ranged from a few minutes to more than three hours; this was independent of the size, volume, and shape of the tablets (69). The effect of the specific gravity of the dosage form also appears to be negligible (64). When single unit formulations are applied with a liquid test meal equivalent to 225 Kcal, gastric emptying of the matrix would not be expected to be grossly delayed, since small meals are removed from the stomach within a relatively short period of time (1–2 hours). However the residence time of such preparations was found to be prolonged to 8 hours or more (65); this probably was related to the fact that subjects were allowed to ingest "low calorie beverages" during the day and to have one or two sandwiches for lunch and supper. These additional snacks obviously were sufficient in some individuals to extend the duration of the digestive period beyond the effects of the small test meal in the morning, and thereby to delay recurrence of fasting motility of the stomach which is required to empty the nondegradable tablet matrix. These data are in accordance with the results obtained with the Heidelberg capsule (60); they demonstrate that gastric retention of single unit products may be highly responsive to **repetitive intake of food** maintaining the digestive motility pattern. This also is in agreement with other observations showing that additional meals at 2 and 4 hours after the initial food intake do prolong the digestive period and postpone removal of nondegradable material from the stomach (80).

   In addition to the influence of meals on gastric residence time of the tablet matrix the release kinetics, the dissolution and stability of the active compound and its transport to the duodenum can be influenced by food; accordingly the systemic availability for various reasons may be altered as compared to fasting drug application.

   Multiple unit controlled release products desintegrating into particles sufficiently small can be handled by the stomach like liquids or liquefied solids; these subunits can leave the stomach practically at any time, during fasting as well as during the digestive period. In the postprandial state there appears to be a size-response-curve between 1.0 and 3.2 mm, with a discrete threshold at 1.4 mm separating different rates of gastric emptying of nonnutritive solid material: 1 mm-objects can leave the stomach as fast as the type of solid food used in these studies; particles up to 3.2 mm in diameter empty more slowly or completely fail to be removed from a food-filled stomach, whereas the material larger than 4 mm consistently is retained until digestion is complete (56). Apart from particle size the volume and the type of liquids used for drug application or the composition of the meal ingested concurrently will contribute to the control of drug delivery to the small intestine. In addition to the gastroduodenal transport of the intact subunits the release of the active ingredient from these small particles may depend on the intragastric or intraintestinal environment and therefore can be affected by a meal.

Both the single unit and the multiple unit controlled release products allow the active compound to become available in the systemic circulation **during** the digestive period. The rate and the extent of systemic availability may be increased or decreased by concurrent food intake as compared to fasting conditions or remain unaffected, as illustrated by the following examples:

Food did not influence the systemic availability of oxprenolol (32), prenalterol (18), and procainamide (74) from certain **single unit products.** Gastric residence time of the procainamide formulation was estimated to be 0.5–2.5 hours when the drug was applied fasting, and 1.5–10 hours when given with a meal; this variability of gastric retention of the nondegradable matrix obviously was irrelevant for the release and the gastroduodenal transport of the active ingredient. In contrast food was shown to enhance the systemic availability of theophylline from a single unit form (34).

Provided the desintegration time of **multiple unit forms** is short, the decomposition to subunits is not rate-limiting for gastric emptying: Application of pellets in a hard gelatine capsule does not retard gastric emptying as compared to predispersing the pellets over the meal; for both ways of drug application, gastric emptying was found to be approximately linear with time, thus following the pattern of liquefied solid food components (68). Apart from brake down to small particles the release of the active ingredient is crucial; by interfering with either of the two processes food can alter the systemic availability of an active compound. For instance food was found to decrease the rate of release of nifedipine (12), resulting in a loss of the biphasic release profile. In addition the extent of systemic availability can be altered; the plasma concentrations of theophylline were decreased when a certain multiple unit controlled release form was coingested with food (34).

Literature reports up to now do not indicate a typical pattern of food effects with either one of the two formulation principles, and therefore do not suggest a general advantage of either dosage form as far as the susceptability to an influence of food is concerned. However part of the data are difficult to interpret, since the papers lack adequate description of the pharmaceutical properties of the products investigated: For example food had no influence (77), substantially affected the systemic availability in children, but not in adults (83), reduced the rate (45, 70) or enhanced the extent (43) of systemic availability of theophylline, when various "sustained" or "extended" release preparations were explored. It remains unclear whether these differences were related to the formulation principle.

The influence of food on the systemic availability of **drugs characterized by a high so-called first pass metabolism** is very complex: The absolute availability is low, when **oral** immediate release preparations are administered fasting, since these compounds are eliminated to a large extent prior to reaching the systemic circulation. Concurrent intake of food enhances the systemic availability, for instance of propranolol, by 50 to 70 per cent (54, 55, 67, 86); a greater effect may be observed when the protein content of the meal is raised (86). Since such drugs are well absorbed when taken fasting, the food-induced increment of plasma concentrations cannot be explained by improvement of absorption, but indicates a reduction of presystemic drug degradation. But this mechanism only operates when immediate release preparations are used, whereas a meal has no effect, when a "sustained release" preparation is applied (10, 46): Presystemic drug elimination is delivery rate dependent; so the **type** of oral formulation determines, whether the systemic availability is increased by concurrent food intake or not. Although the absolute availability is said to be characteristic of a substance rather than a dosage form (98), the data on propranolol demonstrate that at least in the **postprandial** state the **absolute availability may reflect the pharmaceutical properties of a certain drug dosage form.** However the issue of meal-related changes in this type of drugs is even more complicated: As opposed to the **pre**systemic elimination the **systemic** clearance, for instance of propranolol, is enhanced by food (67): As a consequence drug concentrations are lowered by the intake of meal, if propranolol is given **intravenously.** So the **systemic availability shortly after a meal** not only differs as a function of the **rate,** but also as a function of the **route** of drug administration.

3.3 With enteric coated dosage forms again two different formulation principles have to be considered: Single unit enteric coated preparations and multiparticulate systems, which are composed of individually coated subunits.

Single unit enteric coated dosage forms constitute the only type of pharmaceutical preparations, in which the physical properties allow a general prediction of an important effect of food: The **onset** of systemic availability is delayed when these products are coingested with a meal, because the intake of liquid or solid food will inhibit the transport of the **intact** dosage form to the small intestine. Monitoring gastric residence time of the dosage form (by coingestion of a Heidelberg capsule) concurrently with plasma concentrations of the active constituent, for example of acetylsalicylic acid, revealed a close correlation between the time of gastric emptying and the time of onset of systemic availability: Following fasting application of a single unit enteric coated tablet the mean gastric retention of the product was 0.8 hours, associated with a mean lag time of 2.7 hours (61); concurrent intake of a meal on average extended gastric residence time of the formulation to 5.9 hours and the lag time to 7.9 hours. Similar observations were reported for single unit enteric coated tablets of 5-amino-salicylic acid (24). If the delay of onset of drug absorption from single unit enteric coated dosage forms caused by food is unwanted, these products should exclusively be applied on an empty stomach. In addition to extending the lag time food can affect the rate and the extent of systemic availability: for instance both were decreased when an enteric coated acetylsalicylic acid tablet was administered with a meal (7).

Repetitive administration of single unit preparations concurrently with food may result in an intragastric accumulation of several doses, if the digestive period is prolonged beyond the dosage interval; this effect would be associated with irregular drug absorption, time periods uncovered by drugs alternating with overdosing (absorption of more than one dose at a time). In drugs with a low therapeutic range this could imply an increased frequency of toxic drug reactions. Patients with disorders of gastric emptying probably are at particular risk of irregular drug absorption.

In contrast **multiple unit enteric coated formulations** decompose into individually enteric coated subunits within the stomach. If these particles are sufficiently small, they can be delivered to the duodenum during fasting as well as the digestive period. Consequently food intake not necessarily delays the onset of drug absorption, but can prolong gastric residence time of the subunits according to the composition of a meal; however this effect is variable: A meal decreased the extent of systemic availability of digoxin when administered as enteric coated granules (4), but had no effect on acetylsalicylic acid (7). With enteric coated indomethacin pellets only the rate of systemic availability was diminished, whereas the amount of drug absorbed was not influenced (79). So multiple unit enteric coated dosage forms resemble the extended release formulations, whereas single unit enteric coated preparations constitute a different pharmaceutical entity.

4. Standards desirable for controlling the influence of nutrition on pharmaceutical products

In practice presumably all drugs are taken fasting as well as concurrently with food. In order to ensure drug efficacy and safety, information is necessary about meal-related changes of the systemic availability.

"Fasting" drug administration usually implies intake on an empty stomach; therefore no food should be ingested for 12–15 hours prior to dosing. Furthermore fasting drug application implies fasting gastric motility, i.e. a typical pattern of gastric handling of liquids and solids including drugs. This interdigestive motility pattern can be maintained while the stomach contains **non-nutritive** material, such as isotonic saline or nondegradable solid markers, but is disrupted by any type of **nutritive** material (73). Consequently drug intake together with beverages like fruit juice (45) cannot be considered as "fasting" drug application, and cannot be regarded as a valid reference procedure for investigation of the effects of a meal. Since the acidity of gastric contents contributes to the control of gastric emptying (20, 47, 58), intake of liquids stimulating acid secretion like coffee or tea prior to drug administration may alter gastric handling of drugs; this also applies to chewing gum, being as effective in stimulating gastric acid output as food (26).

Changes of the systemic availability resulting from **coingestion of a meal** mostly are unpredictable, because they depend on the pharmaceutical properties of a particular product. Therefore each dosage form has to be investigated separately. In general this will be done in healthy individuals. If the results of these studies are expected to be relevant for drug therapy in patients, they have to be reproducible and representative as well. This will only be possible, if the diet is standardized. Guidelines for performance of biopharmaceutical studies therefore recommend nutrition to be controlled (1, 2, 59, 78, 98).

During assessment of the systemic availability the diet should be **in accordance with modern dietary recommendations for prevention and control of diseases.** These recommendations – **addressing the majority of the western population** – agree in several points, including the advice to reduce total fat intake to 30% of energy or less (36, 66, 89). Therefore a balanced diet containing no more than 30% of fat should be the first joice for biopharmaceutical studies too. Even though the use of high fat meals still is advocated (78), it should be abandonned, because it does not meet adequate nutritional standards. The interest in high fat meals mainly has been based on the assumption of improved drug absorption due to facilitated release and/or dissolution of certain compounds in the presence of fat and bile acids. However it has not been proven that this is the mechanism primarily responsible for a food-induced increase of the systemic availability. Because of its high energy density fat is a potent inhibitor of gastric emptying; therefore the effects of high fat meals could be merely a function of time (prolonged gastric retention of a medicinal product), resulting in release of larger amounts of the active ingredient. Yet extending the duration of the digestive period also can be achieved by means other than increasing the fat content of a meal. Therefore attributing the effects of large meals exclusively to their content of fat may be misleading. To date literature reports do not provide appropriate criteria to differentiate between direct (solubility of the active compound) and indirect (gastric residence time of the dosage form) effects of dietary fat.

Apart from the influence of food on drug absorption the composition of a meal can be relevant for drug elimination too. The data available so far indicate a predominant role of the **protein** content not only for hepatic metabolism, but possibly also for renal excretion of certain compounds (88). These observations provide further evidence that it is not justified to focus primarily on the fat content when assessing the influence of food on the systemic availability of drugs.

Studies should be performed to obtain evidence about the **contribution of**

gastric residence time to food-induced changes of the systemic availability. These investigations should be based on a diet as outlined above (no more than 30% fat). The duration of the digestive period (and thereby gastric retention of drugs) could be varied by **altering** the **digestibility of food,** or the **total amount of energy supplied with a test meal,** or by **meal frequency:** For instance a liquid test meal equivalent to 345–395 Kcal was found to leave the stomach within 139–140 minutes (irrespectively of whether a no-fat meal or a high-fat meal was used! (38)); with test meals equivalent to 500–600 Kcal the digestive period was observed to vary between 3–5 h (48, 60). With larger meals fasting motility will be interrupted for longer periods of time. Solid food mostly has to be reduced in particle size during digestion; decreasing the digestibility, for example by using products rich in dietary fiber, may prolong the time necessary for completion of the digestive process. Additional meals, for instance at 2 to 3 h intervals subsequently to the initial food intake also extend the duration of the digestive period (60, 80), and may delay recurrence of fasting motility to more than 14.5 h. Thereby meal frequency – in addition to the composition of food – can affect gastric retention of drugs.

When **test meals of different composition** are compared with respect to their influence on the systemic availability of drugs (35), no more than one group of nutrients – carbohydrates, fat, protein – should be exchanged at one time. If two or all three components deviate, it is not possible any more to attribute the effects of the meal to one particular constituent, for instance fat. Apart from the absolute amounts of nutrients, the digestibility of food also is relevant for gastric emptying, if conventional products are used. Varying the type of raw products therefore may result in a variable duration of the digestive period, even though the amount of nutrients is kept constant. This is the reason why literature reports in addition to the **estimated** intake of nutrients should precisely describe the amount and the type of food items used for a test meal. In general **nutrient intake** is calculated on the basis of food composition tables; it is uncommon to determine food constituents by chemical analysis. But the composition of the products actually available for preparation of a diet may differ from the average values given in tables; usually these differences remain obscure. Despite of these obvious disadvantages the use of regular food in biopharmaceutical studies should have priority over unusual diets like defined formula diets, because conventional food will allow to generate information on drugs which is more readily applicable to patients. However investigators should be well aware of the limitations of this approach.

The general rule that diet composition in biopharmaceutical studies should meet the standards set for the majority of the population, may be unacceptable with drugs, in which safety in healthy individuals is related to nutrition, for instance antidiabetic compounds. In this case a specified approach may be necessary to ensure safety in healthy volunteers. Further exceptions may be appropriate for investigation of therapeutic agents often combined with a special dietary regimen. For example it might be important to determine the influence of liquid formula diets on drugs used for treatment of inflammatory bowel disease.

Gastric residence time of drugs can differ in males and females (61); this increases the variation of the results within a study. If females are enrolled in biopharmaceutical studies, they should enter the investigation strictly synchronized according to the follicular or luteal phase, since gastric emptying of digestible solids varies with the menstrual cycle (22); otherwise the interindividual variation of food effects will be greater, thus adding to a loss of the discriminating potency of statistical methods.

The characteristics of pharmaceutical products worked out in healthy individuals are likely to be representative for patients, unless drug absorption, distribution, or elimination is modified by the underlying disease. When oral dosage forms are used, **disorders of gastric emptying** can be of primary importance with respect to an alteration of the systemic availability; this is relevant for therapeutic drug application as well as for biopharmaceutical studies. Deviations of gastric motor function may involve emptying of liquids or solids or both. Impaired gastric emptying can be due to mechanical obstruction of the gastric outlet, for instance by malignancies or bulbar scarring, or due to postsurgical defects (25, 41, 50, 51, 52) or other conditions associated with abnormal gastric motility (5, 30, 53, 58, 62, 63, 93). These include quite heterogeneous disorders, chronic as well as acute intermittent or recurrent diseases such as diabetes mellitus, scleroderma, central nervous system lesions, spinal cord injury (76), dystrophia myotonica (29), peptic ulcer disease (96, 97), sepsis, pancreatitis, viral gastroenteritis, migraine attacks (84), zoster thoracalis (37), or malnutrition in anorexia nervosa. Absence of the "ileal brake" following distal small bowel resection also can affect the rate of gastric emptying (47). Furthermore certain drugs like opiates, anticholinergics, tricyclic antidepressants, β-adrenergic agonists (58), and radiation therapy of the abdomen (44) can induce abnormalities of gastric motor function.

Even severe impairment of gastric emptying can remain asymptomatic and undetected (93); in patients who indeed do present with symptoms, the disorder is likely to be more pronounced than in patients who do not complain of problems (82). At least in patients who are symptomatic, gastric motor function should be taken into account in drug prescription: The dosage form should be carefully selected according to the type and extent of gastric emptying disorder. Maximum care is required when drugs are given **repetitively** in patients with delayed gastric emptying. Prolonged retention of the dosage form may not be hazardous, if the active ingredient is released to a sufficient extent within the stomach and can be transported to the duodenum during the digestive period; however it could be harmful with single unit formulations retaining all or most of the active compound: Patients would be at increased risk of irregular drug absorption, if gastric residence time of the dosage form was prolonged beyond the dosage interval. This could happen for instance in diabetic patients with gastric stasis, who are advised to have frequent small meals, thus extending their digestive periods in a variable and unpredictable way. Furthermore single unit dosage forms can cause problems in patients with permanent gastric outlet obstruction or absence of phase 3 contraction waves, since these patients may not be able at all to remove nondegradable material from their stomach. Lack of phase 3 activity is assumed to contribute to "bezoar" formation (53, 58, 62, 63, 93). Apart from phyto- and trichobezoars "pharmacobezoars" also are known to occur: For instance enteric coated acetylsalicylic acid preparations (6), "slow release" theophylline (11) and an ion exchange resin (42) have been reported to result in intragastric conglomeration.

In older age groups gastric motor function can be altered without an underlying disease: Impaired gastric emptying of both indigestible solids (lack of phase 3 activity in the fasting state [47]) and digestible solids (prolongation of the digestive period [93, 94]) is observed. Therefore single unit dosage forms do not appear to be appropriate pharmaceutical formulations for drug treatment in geriatric patients, even though these preparations are recommended for reduction of the frequency of dosing.

With respect to the problems possibly arising from the use of controlled release and enteric coated products it is desirable to include details on the pharmaceutical formulation into the product information, with special reference to the differentiation between single unit and multiple unit preparations. This information is mandatory for the physician in care to select individually safe drug dosage forms.

5. Literature

(1) APV – Arbeitsgemeinschaft für pharmazeutische Verfahrenstechnik, Fachgruppe "Biopharmazie". Untersuchungen zur Bioverfügbarkeit, Bioäquivalenz. APV-Richtlinie. Pharm. Ind. 49, 704–707 (1987)

(2) APV – International Association for Pharmaceutical Technology, Working Group "Biopharmacy". Studies on bioavailability and bioequivalence. AVP Guideline. Drugs Made in Germany 30, 161–166 (1987)

(3) Bauer, K. H., Frömming, K. H., Führer, C.: Pharmazeutische Technologie. Georg Thieme Verlag Stuttgart (1986)

(4) Bergdahl, B., Bogentoft, C., Jonsson, U. E., Magnusson, J. O.: Fasting and postprandial absorption of digoxin from a microencapsu-

lated formulation. Eur. J. Clin. Pharmacol. 25, 207–210 (1983)

(5) Blum, A. L., Sonnenberg, A., Siewert, R.: Motilitätsstörungen von Magen und Pylorus. Internist 20, 10–17 (1979)

(6) Bogacz, K., Caldron, P.: Enteric-coated aspirin bezoar: Elevation of serum salicylate level by barium study. Am. J. Med. 83, 783–786 (1987)

(7) Bogentoft, C., Carlsson, I., Ekenved, G., Magnusson, A.: Influence of food on the absorption of acetylsalicylic acid from enteric-coated dosage forms. Eur. J. Clin. Pharmacol. 14, 351–355 (1978)

(8) Burgess, P., Hall, R. I., Bateman, D. N., Johnston, I. D. A.: Antipyrine clearance dur-

ing total parenteral nutrition in man. Br. J. Clin. Pharmacol. *20*, 253P–254P (1985)

(9) Bury, K. D., Jambunathan, G.: Effects of elemental diets on gastric emptying and gastric secretion in man. Am. J. Surg. *127*, 59–64 (1974)

(10) Byrne, A. J., McNeil, J. J., Harrison, P. M., Louis, W., Tonkin, A. M., McLean, A. J.: Stable oral availability of sustained release propranolol when co-administered with hydralazine or food: Evidence implicating substrate delivery rate as a determinant of presystemic drug interactions. Br. J. Clin. Pharmacol. *17*, 45S–50S (1984)

(11) Cereda, J. M., Scott, J., Quigley, E. M. M.: Endoscopic removal of pharmacobezoar of slow release theophylline. Br. med. J. *293*, 1143 (1986)

(12) Challenor, V., Waller, D. G., Gruchy, B. S., Renwick, A. G., George, C. F., McMurdo, E. T., McEwen, J.: The effects of food and posture on the pharmacokinetics of a biphasic release preparation of nifedipine. Br. J. Clin. Pharmacol. *22*, 565–570 (1986)

(13) Clements, J. A., Heading, R. C., Nimmo, V. S., Prescott, L. F.: Kinetics of acetaminophen absorption and gastric emptying in man. Clin. Pharmacol. Ther. *24*, 420–431 (1978)

(14) Collins, P. J., Horowitz, M., Cook, D. J., Harding, P. E., Shearman, D. J. C.: Gastric emptying in normal subjects – a reproducible technique using a single scintillation camera and computer system. Gut *24*, 1117–1125 (1983)

(15) Conney, A. H., Pantuck, E. J., Hsiao, K. C., Garland, W. A., Anderson, K. E., Alvarez, A. P., Kappas, A.: Enhanced phenacetin metabolism in human subjects fed charcoal-broiled beef. Clin. Pharmacol. Ther. *20*, 633–642 (1976)

(16) Cortot, A., Phillips, S. F., Malagelada, J. R.: Gastric emptying of lipids after ingestion of an homogenized meal. Gastroenterology *76*, 939–944 (1979)

(17) Cortot, A., Phillips, S. F., Malagelada, J. R.: Gastric emptying of lipids after ingestion of a solid-liquid meal in humans. Gastroenterology *80*, 922–927 (1981)

(18) Dahlström, U., Graffner, C., Jonsson, U., Hoffmann, K. J., Karlsson, E., Lagerström, P. O.: Pharmacokinetics of prenalterol after single and multiple administration of controlled release tablets to patients with congestive heart failure. Eur. J. Clin. Pharmacol. *24*, 495–502 (1983)

(19) Dickson, C. J., Schwartzman, M. S., Bertino, J. S., Jr.: Factors affecting aminoglycoside disposition: Effects of circadian rhythm and dietary protein intake on gentamycin pharmacokinetics. Clin. Pharmacol. Ther. *39*, 325–328 (1986)

(20) Dooley, C. P., Reznick, J. B., Valenzuela, J. E.: Variations in gastric and duodenal motility during gastric emptying of liquid meals in humans. Gastroenterology *87*, 1114–1119 (1984)

(21) Food and Drug Administration: Rules and regulations. § 320.1 Definitions. Federal Register *42*, 1618 (1977)

(22) Gill, R. C., Murphy, P. D., Hooper, H. R., Bowes, K. L., Kingma, Y. J.: Effect of the menstrual cycle on gastric emptying. Digestion *36*, 168–174 (1987)

(23) Grimes, D. S., Goddard, J.: Gastric emptying of wholemeal and white bread. Gut *18*, 725–729 (1977)

(24) Hardy, J. G., Healey, J. N. C., Lee, S. W., Reynolds, J. R.: Gastrointestinal transit of an enteric-coated delayed-release 5-aminosalicylic acid tablet. Aliment. Pharmacol. Ther. *1*, 209–216 (1987)

(25) Heading, R. C., Tothill, P., McLoughlin, G. P., Shearman, D. J. C.: Gastric emptying rate measurement in man. A double isotope scanning technique for simultaneous study of liquid and solid components of a meal. Gastroenterology *71*, 45–50 (1976)

(26) Helman, C. A.: Chewing gum is as effective as food in stimulating cephalic phase gastric secretion. Am. J. Gastroenterol. *83*, 640–642 (1988)

(27) Holgate, A. M., Read, N. W.: Effect of ileal infusion of intralipid on gastrointestinal transit, ileal flow rate and carbohydrate absorption in humans after ingestion of a liquid meal. Gastroenterology *88*, 1005–1011 (1985)

(28) Holt, S., Reid, J., Taylor, T. V., Tothill, P., Heading, R. C.: Gastric emptying of solids in man. Gut *23*, 292–296 (1982)

(29) Horowitz, M., Maddox, A., Maddern, G. J., Wishart, J., Collins, P. J., Shearman, D. J. C.: Gastric and esophageal emptying in dystrophia myotonica. Gastroenterology *92*, 570–577 (1987)

(30) Hunt, J. N.: Mechanisms and disorders of gastric emptying. Ann. Rev. Med. *34*, 219–229 (1983)

(31) Hunt, J. N., Stubbs, D. F.: The volume and energy content of meals are determinants of gastric emptying. J. Physiol. (London) *245*, 209–225 (1975)

(32) John, V. A., Smith, S. E.: Influence of food intake on plasma oxprenolol concentrations following oral administration of conventional and Oros preparations. Br. J. Clin. Pharmacol. *19*, 191S–195S (1985)

(33) Kappas, A., Anderson, K. E., Conney, A. H., Alvarez, A. P.: Influence of dietary protein and carbohydrate on antipyrine and theophylline metabolism in man. Clin. Pharmacol. Ther. 20, 643–653 (1976)

(34) Karim, A., Burns, T., Wearley, L., Streicher, J., Palmer, M.: Food-induced changes in theophylline absorption from controlled-release formulations. Part I. Substantial increased and decreased absorption with Uniphyl tablets and Theo-Dur Sprinkle. Clin. Pharmacol. Ther. 38, 77–83 (1985)

(35) Karim, A., Burns, T., Janky, D., Hurwitz, A.: Food-induced changes in theophylline absorption from controlled-release formulations. Part II. Importance of meal composition and dosing time relative to meal intake in assessing changes in absorption. Clin. Pharmacol. Ther. 38, 642–647 (1985)

(36) Kasper, H.: Ernährungsmedizin und Diätetik. 6. Auflage, Urban und Schwarzenberg. München (1987)

(37) Kebede, D., Barthel, J. S., Singh, A.: Transient gastroparesis associated with cutaneous herpes zoster. Dig. Dis. Sci. 32, 318–322 (1987)

(38) Kellow, J. E., Borody, T. J., Phillips, S. F., Tucker, R. L., Haddad, A. C.: Human interdigestive motility: variations in patterns from esophagus to colon. Gastroenterology 91, 386–395 (1986)

(39) Kelly, K. A.: Gastric emptying of liquids and solids: Roles of proximal and distal stomach. Am. J. Physiol. 239, G71–G76 (1980)

(40) Krishnaswamy, K., Kalamegham, R., Naidu, N. A.: Dietary influences on the kinetics of antipyrine and aminopyrine in human subjects. Br. J. Clin. Pharmacol. 17, 139–146 (1984)

(41) Kroop, H. W., Long, W. B., Alavi, A., Hansell, J. R.: Effect of water and fat on gastric emptying of solid meals. Gastroenterology 77, 997–1000 (1979)

(42) Künzel, W., Meissner, D.: Bezoar aus Partikeln des Kationenaustauschers Elutit^R. Z. Klin. Med. 41, 1483–1484 (1986)

(43) Lagas, M., Jonkman, J. H. G.: Influence of food on the rate and extent of absorption of theophylline after single dose oral administration of a controlled release tablet. Int. J. Clin. Pharmacol. 23, 424–426 (1985)

(44) Layer, P., Demol, P., Hotz, J., Goebell, H.: Gastroparesis after radiation. Successful treatment with carbachol. Dig. Dis. Sci. 31, 1377–1380 (1986)

(45) Leeds, N. H., Gal, P., Purohit, A. A., Walter, J. B.: Effect of food on the bioavailability and pattern of release of a sustained-release theophylline tablet. J. Clin. Pharmacol. 22, 196–200 (1982)

(46) Liedholm, H., Melander, A.: Concomitant food intake can increase the bioavailability of propranolol by transient inhibition of its presystemic primary conjugation. Clin. Pharmacol. Ther. 40, 29–36 (1986)

(47) Lübke, H. J., Wienbeck, M.: Gastrointestinale Motilität und enterale Resorption beeinflussen sich gegenseitig. Klinikarzt 14, 25–36 (1985)

(48) Lübke, H. J., Winkelmann, R. S., Erckenbrecht, J. F., Wienbeck, M.: Einfluß von L-Tryptophan auf die intestinale Nüchternmotilität und auf die Dünndarmtransitzeit beim Menschen. Z. Gastroenterologie 25, 701–708 (1987)

(49) Malagelada, J. R., Go, V. L. W., Summerskill, W. H. J.: Different gastric, pancreatic, and biliary responses to solid-liquid or homogenized meals. Dig. Dis. Sci. 24, 101–110 (1979)

(50) Malagelada, J. R., Rees, W. D. W., Mazzotta, L. J., Go, V. L. W.: Gastric motor abnormalities in diabetic and postvagotomy gastroparesis: Effect of metoclopramide and bethanechol. Gastroenterology 78, 286–293 (1980)

(51) Mayer, E. A., Thomson, J. B., Jehn, D., Reedy, T., Elashoff, J., Meyer, J. H.: Gastric emptying and sieving of solid food and pancreatic and biliary secretion after solid meals in patients with truncal vagotomy and antrectomy. Gastroenterology 83, 184–192 (1982)

(52) Mayer, E. A., Thomson, J. B., Jehn, D., Reedy, T., Elashoff, J., Deveny, C., Meyer, J. H.: Gastric emptying and sieving of solid food and pancreatic and biliary secretions after solid meals in patients with nonresective ulcer surgery. Gastroenterology 87, 1264–1271 (1984)

(53) McCallum, R. W.: Gastric emptying disorders. Tests and treatments. Postgrad. Med. 81, 67–76 (1987)

(54) McLean, A. J., Isbister, C., Bobik, A., Dudley, F. J.: Reduction of first-pass hepatic clearance of propranolol by food. Clin. Pharmacol. Ther. 30, 31–34 (1981)

(55) Melander, A., Danielson, K., Schersten, B., Wahlin, E.: Enhancement of the bioavailability of propranolol and metoprolol by food. Clin. Pharmacol. Ther. 22, 108–112 (1977)

(56) Meyer, J. H., Elashoff, J., Porter-Fink, V., Dressman, J., Amidon, G. L.: Human postprandial gastric emptying of 1-3-millimeter spheres. Gastroenterology 94, 1315–1325 (1988)

(57) Miller, L. J., Malagelada, J. R., Taylor, W. F., Go, V. L. W.: Intestinal control of human

postprandial gastric function: The role of components of jejunoileal chyme in regulating gastric secretion and gastric emptying. Gastroenterology 80, 763–769 (1981)

(58) Minami, H., McCallum, R. W.: The physiology and pathophysiology of gastric emptying in humans. Gastroenterology 86, 1592–1610 (1984)

(59) Ministry of Health and Welfare, Scientific Research, Tokyo, Japan: Guidelines for the application for product approval of oral sustained release dosage forms; draft (1987)

(60) Mojaverian, P., Ferguson, R. K., Vlasses, P. H., Rocci, M. L., Jr., Oren, A., Fix, J. A., Caldwell, L. J., Gardner, C.: Estimation of gastric residence time of the Heidelberg capsule in humans: Effect of varying food composition. Gastroenterology 89, 392–397 (1985)

(61) Mojaverian, P., Rocci, M. L., Jr., Conner, D. P., Abrams, W. B., Vlasses, P. H.: Effect of food on the absorption of enteric-coated aspirin: Correlation with gastric residence time. Clin. Pharmacol. Ther. 41, 11–17 (1987)

(62) Müller-Lissner, S. A.: Gestörte Magenentleerung. In: Therapie gastrointestinaler Motilitätsstörungen. Eds.: M. Wienbeck, J. R. Siewert. Edition Medizin, Verlag Chemie, Weinheim, pp 31–46 (1984)

(63) Müller-Lissner, S.: Die normale Magenentleerung und ihre Störungen. Leber Magen Darm 16, 11–19 (1986)

(64) Müller-Lissner, S. A., Blum, A. L.: The effect of specific gravity and eating on gastric emptying of slow-release capsules. N. Engl. J. Med. 304, 1365–1366 (1981)

(65) Müller-Lissner, S. A., Will, N., Müller-Duysing, W., Heinzel, F., Blum, A. L.: Schwimmkapseln mit langsamer Wirkstoffabgabe. Dtsch. Med. Wochenschr. 106, 1143–1147 (1981)

(66) Nestle, M.: Nutrition in clinical practice. Jones Medical Publications, Greenbrae (1985)

(67) Olanoff, L. S., Walle, T., Cowart, T. D., Walle, U. K., Oexmann, M. J., Conradi, E. C.: Food effects on propranolol systemic and oral clearance: Support for a blood flow hypothesis. Clin. Pharmacol. Ther. 40, 408–414 (1986)

(68) O'Reilly, S., Wilson, C. G., Hardy, J. G.: The influence of food on the gastric emptying of multiparticulate dosage forms. Int. J. Pharmac. 34, 213–216 (1987)

(69) Park, H. M., Chernish, S. M., Rosenek, B. D., Brunell, R. L., Hargrove, B., Wellman, H. N.: Gastric emptying of enteric-coated tablets. Dig. Dis. Sci. 29, 207–212 (1984)

(70) Pedersen, S.: Delay in the absorption rate of theophylline from a sustained release theophylline preparation caused by food. Br. J. Clin. Pharmacol. 12, 904–905 (1981)

(71) Read, N. W.: The control of gastrointestinal transit by luminal nutrients. In: Intestinal absorption and secretion. Eds.: E. Skadhauge, K. Heintze. MTP Press Ltd., Lancaster, pp 153–160 (1984)

(72) Read, N. W., McFarlane, A., Kinsman, R. I., Bates, T. E., Blackhall, N. W., Farrar, G. B. J., Hall, J. C., Moss, G., Morris, A. P., O'Neill, B., Welch, I., Lee, Y., Bloome, S. R.: Effect of infusion of nutrient solutions into the ileum on gastrointestinal transit and plasma levels of neurotensin and enteroglucagon. Gastroenterology 86, 274–280 (1984)

(73) Rees, W. D. W., Malagelada, J. R., Miller, L. J., Go, V. L. W.: Human interdigestive and postprandial gastrointestinal motor and gastrointestinal hormone patterns. Dig. Dis. Sci. 27, 321–329 (1982)

(74) Rocci, M. L., Mojaverian, P., Davis, R. J., Ferguson, R. K., Vlasses, P. H.: Food-induced gastric retention and absorption of sustained-release procainamide. Clin. Pharmacol. Ther. 42, 45–49 (1987)

(75) Ruppin, H., Bar-Meir, S., Soergel, K. H., Wood, C. M.: Effects of liquid formula diets on proximal gastrointestinal function. Dig. Dis. Sci. 26, 202–207 (1981)

(76) Segal, J. L., Milne, N., Brunnemann, S. R., Lyons, K. P.: Metoclopramide-induced normalization of impaired gastric emptying in spinal cord injury. Am. J. Gastroenterol. 82, 1143–1148 (1987)

(77) Sips, A. P., Edelbroek, P. M., Kulstad, S., de Wolff, F. A., Dijkman, J. H.: Food does not effect in bioavailability of theophylline from Theolin Retard^R. Eur. J. Clin. Pharmacol. 26, 405–407 (1984)

(78) Skelly, J. P., Barr, W. H., Benet, L. Z., Doluisio, J. T., Goldberg, A. H., Levy, G., Lowenthal, D. T., Robinson, J. R., Shah, V. P., Temple, R. J., Yacobi, A.: Report of the workshop on controlled release dosage forms: Issues and controversies (1985)

(79) Skinhøj, A., Bechgard, H., Chasseaud, L. F., Brodie, R. R., Sharman, J. M., Taylor, T., Hunter, J. O.: The influence of food and repeated dosing on the bioavailability of indomethacin from a multiple-units controlled release formulation. Int. J. Clin. Pharmacol. 22, 557–561 (1984)

(80) Smith, H. J., Feldman, M.: Influence of food and marker length on gastric emptying of indigestible radiopaque markers in healthy humans. Gastroenterology 91, 1452–1455 (1986)

(81) Smith, J. L., Jiang, C. L., Hunt, J. N.: Intrinsic emptying pattern of the human stomach. Am. J. Physiol. *246*, R959–R962 (1984)

(82) Smout, A. J. P. M., Akkermans, L. M. A., Roelofs, J. M. M., Pasma, F. G., Oei, H. Y., Wittebol, P.: Gastric emptying and postprandial symptoms after Billroth II resection. Surgery *101*, 27–34 (1987)

(83) Steffensen, G., Pedersen, S.: Food induced changes in theophylline absorption from a once-a-day theophylline product. Br. J. Clin. Pharmacol. *22*, 571–577 (1986)

(84) Tokola, R. A., Neuvonen, P. J.: Effect of migraine attacks on paracetamol absorption. Br. J. Clin. Pharmacol. *18*, 867–871 (1984)

(85) Tranvouez, J. L., Lerebours, E., Chretien, P., Fouin-Fortunet, H., Colin, R.: Hepatic antipyrine metabolism in malnourished patients: Influence of the type of malnutrition and course after nutritional rehabilitation. Am. J. Clin. Nutr. *41*, 1257–1264 (1985)

(86) Walle, T., Fagan, T. C., Walle, K., Oexmann, M. J., Conradi, E. C., Gaffney, T. E.: Food – induced increase in propranolol bioavailability – relationship to protein and effects on metabolites. Clin. Pharmacol. Ther. *30*, 790–795 (1981)

(87) Walter-Sack, I.: The influence of nutrition on the systemic availability of drugs. Part I: Drug absorption. Klin. Wochenschr. *65*, 927–935 (1987)

(88) Walter-Sack, I.: The influence of nutrition on the systemic availability of drugs. Part II: Drug metabolism and renal excretion. Klin. Wochenschr. *65*, 1062–1072 (1987)

(89) Walter-Sack, I.: Recommendations for controlling the effects of nutrition during assessment of the systemic availability of drugs. Klin. Wochenschr. *65*, 1109–1112 (1987)

(90) Walter-Sack, I., de Vries, J. X., Ittensohn, A., Kohlmeier, M., Weber, E.: Benzbromarone disposition and uricosuric action; evidence for hydroxilation instead of debromination to benzarone. Klin. Wochenschr. *66*, 160–166 (1988)

(91) Walter-Sack, I,, Luckow, V., Guserle, R., Weber, E.: Untersuchungen zur relativen Bioverfügbarkeit von Paracetamol nach Gabe von festen und flüssigen oralen Zubereitungen sowie rektalen Applikationsformen. Arzneim. Forsch./Drug. Res. (1989)

(92) Walter-Sack, I. E., de Vries, J. X., Nickel, B., Stenzhorn, G., Weber, E.: The influence of different balanced test meals and different pharmaceutical formulations on the systemic availability of paracetamol, gallbladder size, and blood glucose (accepted for publication). Int. J. Clin. Pharmacol.

(93) Wegener, M., Schaffstein, J., Börsch, G.: Physiologie und Pathophysiologie der Magenentleerung. Med. Klinik *83*, 335–341 (1988)

(94) Wegener, M., Börsch, G., Schaffstein, J., Lüth, I., Rickels, R., Ricken, D.: Effect of ageing on the gastro-intestinal transit of a lactulose-supplemented mixed solid-liquid meal in humans. Digestion *39*, 40–46 (1988)

(95) Wienbeck, M., Erckenbrecht, J. F., Enck, P.: Neue Entwicklungen in der gastrointestinalen Motilität. Internist *27*, 714–722 (1986)

(96) Wienbeck, M., Lübke, H. J.: Motilität und peptisches Ulkus – mögliche pathogenetische Verbindungen. Z. Gastroenterologie *25*, Suppl. 3, 64–68 (1987)

(97) Williams, M. S., Elashoff, J., Meyer, J. H.: Gastric emptying of liquids in normal subjects and in patients with healed duodenal ulcer disease. Dig. Dis. Sci. *31*, 943–952 (1986)

(98) World Health Organisation, Regional Office for Europe: Guidelines for the investigation of bioavailability. Revised draft (1986)

VIII. In vitro-Dissolution Testing of Oral Controlled Release Products

Martin Siewert, Eschborn

Summary

The importance of in vitro-dissolution testing for the assessment of the pharmaceutical quality of controlled release dosage forms is emphasized. Different test models and their suitabilities are discussed. Relevant parameters of the experimental conditions are e.g. pH, surface tension, ionic strength. Their possible interaction with the physico-chemical properties of the drug substance and the galenical formulation are described.

A validation of an individual in vitro-model once set up requires parallel in vitro- and in vivo-studies. In certain cases, where biopharmaceutical characteristics of different formulations are well known, a validation can be successfully performed without bioavailability studies to prove the plausibility of an in vitro-test system.

For establishing valid specifications and acceptance-criteria for the in vitro-dissolution tests of oral controlled release dosage forms pharmacokinetic properties of the drug substance and the galenical dosage form as well as the pharmacodynamic characteristics of the active substances are to be well known.

Different approaches for a standardization of the in vitro-dissolution tests of controlled release dosage forms, such as the USP-Policy on Modified-release Dosage Forms and the Japanese Guidelines for the Application for Product Approval of Oral Sustained Release Dosage Forms are critically discussed.

1. Application of in vitro-dissolution tests

Controlled release products are characterized by a modified, extended and/or delayed dissolution of the active constituent, a process which accounts for the importance of in vitro-dissolution tests within the testing and assessment of their pharmaceutical quality.

The appropriate tests are used within galenical development, quality assurance of preparations for clinical trials, stability testing and the compilation of documentation for registration. Once the preparation has been introduced on to the market, in vitro-dissolution tests are used for the evaluation of the relevance of changes in the formulation, different manufacturing stages or production sites and are, in addition, an important component of the quality assurance system and an essential prerequisite for bioavailability and bioequivalence studies.

For the comprehensive evaluation of the biopharmaceutical properties of a controlled release drug very extensive in vitro-dissolution tests, which are usually carried out under various test conditions, possibly with different test models, are necessary within the different steps of galenical development. However, this comprehensive test programme is reduced to a single test procedure with adequate discriminating potency for the purposes of quality control for batch release.

Nowadays, the in vitro-dissolution test is the most important test criterion in the comparative assessment of commercial controlled release drugs with the same active substance ("generics"), e. g. by independent institutions. Difficulties can arise as regards the stipulation of suitable test conditions, assessment criteria and particularly a requirement profile, because the procedure usually entails the comparative testing of preparations from different manufacturers and consequently also different dosage forms and different galenical principles. The reliability of data obtained solely in vitro is often restricted by the question of the therapeutic importance of differences determined in the in vitro-dissolution profiles of the active substance. However, the fundamental importance of in vitro-dissolution tests for controlled release preparations is apparent from the fact that the aim of the development of these dosage forms is to make the dissolution of the active substance represent the rate-determining pharmacokinetic step in vivo.

2. Test methods and conditions

There are no legally binding regulations, specific to controlled-release dosage forms, concerning the selection of apparatus and experimental conditions for in vitro-dissolution tests. The paddle or rotating basket model described in USP XXI, the European and other Pharmacopoeias is a simple, robust and adequately standardized apparatus which is used virtually the world over and thus is characterized by the most experimental experience. It is because of these advantages that the paddle and rotating basket apparatus is recommended in various guidelines for the in vitro-dissolution testing of controlled release preparations, e. g. the FIP-Guidelines for Dissolution Testing of Solid

Oral Products (1), the USP Policy on Modified-release Dosage Forms (2) and the Japanese Guidelines for the Application for Product Approval of Oral Sustained Release Dosage Forms (3).

However, because of the 'single container' nature of the paddle apparatus experimental difficulties can arise in terms of a change in pH or a (partial) change in the test medium during an investigation, a number of sparingly soluble drugs and dosage forms that tend to (initial) floating, particularly aerophilic multiple unit forms. The flow-through cell according to DAC 1986 (4), which was recommended by the FIP Guidelines (1) and has now been proposed for the European Pharmacopoeia, has distinct advantages in these critical cases (5).

Moreover, a number of alternative dissolution models that differ from the pharmacopeial test methods are given in the literature for the dissolution testing of modified release dosage forms. These include for example a modified disintegration tester known as BIO-DIS apparatus which was found suitable for the in vitro-testing of especially a number of pellet preparations (6). Other apparatuses used are the dissolution model according to Stricker (7), the rotating flask model Resotest (8) which is based on the principle of a rotary evaporator, a rotating flow-through cell (9) and other computer-controlled flow-through models (10). In vivo/in vitro-correlations have been

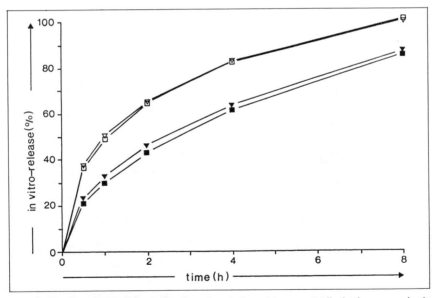

Fig. 1: Influence of agitation on in vitro-dissolution of two controlled release products
Diltiazem (-■- 50 rpm; -▼- 100 rpm)
Metoprolol (-□- 50 rpm; -▽- 100 rpm)

elaborated with these test models for a number of drugs and consequently their suitability for the assessment of the quality of these controlled release preparations was demonstrated. However these methods are by no means as widely used as the pharmacopeial standard methods and experience of them is thus more restricted.

Once a suitable apparatus has been selected, it is crucially important to stipulate the experimental conditions for in vitro-dissolution testing. Since, with controlled-release preparations, the dissolution rate of the active substance is determined by the galenical formulation and should be influenced as little as possible by external circumstances, agitation of the test medium, stirring speed or flow rate, often has only a slight effect on the rate of dissolution (Fig. 1) except in the case of eroding or swelling galenical formulations.

In the case of controlled release forms with pH-dependent dissolution characteristics of the active substance, increased inter- an intraindividual variabilitiy is to be expected as a matter of course during drug therapy; this is due to the patient's age, sex, individually varying and sometimes fluctuating pH conditions in the gastrointestinal tract, eating habits and the time of day that the drug is taken. Thus for a qualified assessment of the biopharmaceutical properties of controlled release drugs it is essential to include a pH-profile of

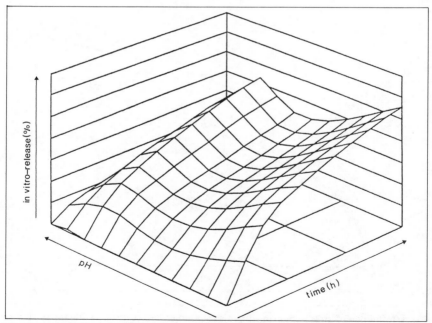

Fig. 2: Topographical dissolution characterization as a function of time and pH (From Skelly, J. et al., ref. 11).

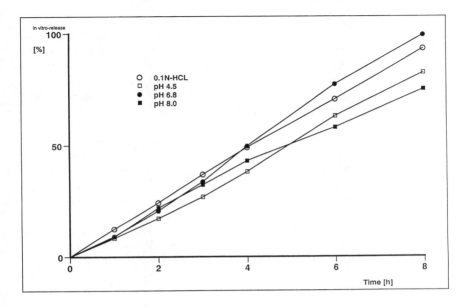

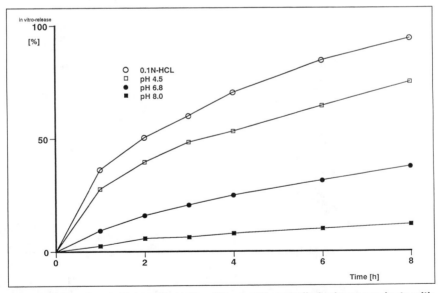

Fig. 3: In vitro-dissolution profiles of two Verapamil controlled release products with pH-independent (upper profiles) and pH-dependent (lower profiles) drug release characteristics

the in vitro-dissolution rates (Fig. 2). Furthermore, in the interests of consistent therapy every effort should be made to develop a formulation with dissolution characteristics that are as far as possible independent of pH (Fig. 3).

Thus when selecting and specifying a certain test medium the greatest importance should be attached to establishing a suitable pH. The physicochemical properties of the drug, particularly its acid/base-properties and possibly the pH-dependency of the release characteristics of the galenical formulation should be taken into account.

In view of the frequent fluctuations in pH values and the absence of buffer capacity, water should not be selected as the test medium for the dissolution testing of controlled release drugs unless the dosage form in question is a galenical formulation releasing independently of pH a drug that also dissociates irrespective of pH. Otherwise widely varying results, which make an assessment of the in vitro-dissolution characteristics and in particular a comparative assessment of preparations with the same active substance impossible, must be expected if water is used for dissolution testing (Fig. 4).

The surface tension of the test medium is another important criterion especially for aerophilic controlled release dosage forms, e.g. many pellets or micromatrices. The poor wettability of these preparations can also yield inconclusive results or marked variations in the measured data (Fig. 5). Wet-

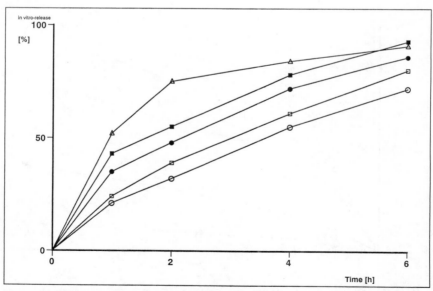

Fig. 4: Mean (n = 6) in vitro-dissolution profiles of five dissolution tests of one batch of a Theophylline controlled release product with pH-dependent drug release characteristics performed in five different weeks using demineralized water as test medium

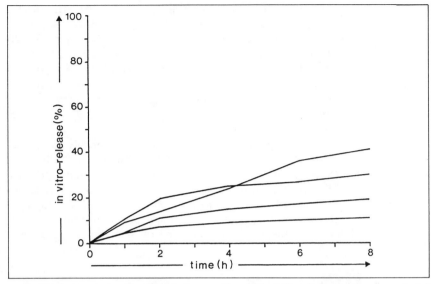

Fig. 5: Mean (n = 6) in vitro-dissolution profiles of four dissolution tests of one batch of Nifedipine controlled release pellets with poor wettability and aerophilic character

ting agents are added in certain cases in order to prevent these critical effects. But surfactants should not be used routinely for the in vitro-dissolution testing of controlled release drugs, because they often restrict the discriminating ability of the test model in question.

With a number of controlled release preparations, e. g. those based on an ion exchange-system, the effect of the ionic strength and the nature of the compensating ion in buffered systems must be monitored and taken into account accordingly when specifying the test medium. In the case of depot systems where the active ingredient is embedded in a fatty substance the addition of lipases to break down the matrix enzymatically has proved advantageous in a number of examples.

The paddle apparatus with a well defined medical liquid food as the test medium has been used successfully (12) for tests where the dissolution rates may depend on food components. It was also helpful, for a correlation of the interaction with food constituents in vivo and in vitro, that the same liquid can also be administered in parallel pharmacokinetic studies in vivo.

In view of the many test models used and the various parameters influencing experimental conditions, it is understandable that proposals aimed at the standardization of dissolution testing of controlled release drugs would be welcomed both by users such as pharmaceutical manufacturers and by the authorities responsible for registration and inspection. On the other hand, because of the marked variations in the physico-chemical properties of the different drugs and the considerable galenical differences between the properties of controlled release formulations, standardization of this type is hardly likely to be very successful or would only succeed in a few individual aspects. A critical examination to establish whether published proposals are correct in all respects is therefore called for. Thus in view of the parameter of the pH value discussed above, the standardization of the test medium to 500–1000 ml water (case 1) in the USP Policy on Modified-Release Dosage Forms (Fig. 6) must be strictly rejected.

The Japanese registration guidelines (3) pursue the scientifically more justifiable route of constructing a test system for the assessment of the in vitro-dissolution characteristics of controlled release forms (Fig. 7). The specification of the detailed test conditions is however left to the applicant, taking account of the properties of the substance, the pharmacokinetics of the drug in question and the characteristics of the specific galenical formulation. The Japanese guidelines can therefore also be used outside the scope of their

---

1. Apparatus
   USP XXI App. I or II. Alternative equipment only if it can be shown that neither App. I nor App. II can be used to characterize a product, or provided that such an alternative method has been validated relative to one specifying an official apparatus.

2. Test conditions (case one)*
   500 to 1000 ml of water as test medium; 100 rpm (App. I) or 50 rpm (App. II)

3. Requirements (case one)*
   $Q_{0.25}$: 20 to 50 % at 0.25 dosing intervals
   $Q_{0.50}$: 45 to 75 % at 0.50 dosing intervals
   $Q_{1.00}$: not less than 75 % at 1.00 dosing intervals

   *Exceptions:
   Case two: Applies where the chemistry or physical properties of the drug or formulations do not allow workable application of case one, or the drug is actually released over a time period less than the dosing interval.

   Case three: Applies where the chemistry or physical properties of the drug formulations among a group of products from different manufacturers differ to such an extent that a single selection of a dissolution test, times, and specifications is not acceptable.

Fig. 6: USP-Policy on Modified-release Dosage Forms (Summary from ref. 2).

A. Release Characteristics	B. Specifications for the Dissolution Test
* The rate of release should be determined in vitro under as many conditions as possible.	* The rate of release and the tolerable range of the release rate cannot be standardized in general.
* The release of the active ingredient should be evaluated at three levels of pH, such as 1.2, 4.0, and 6.8.	* Convenient times to collect sample solutions should be set so that 30 $\pm$10 %, 50 $\pm$10 %, and 90 $\pm$10 % of the labelled amount is released.
* Agitation rates should vary more than two levels (Paddle: 50, 100, 200 rpm)	* Measured values of all six samples collected at each specified time should be within the tolerable range, or not more than two of twelve samples are outside.
* It is desirable to conduct several tests using different apparatuses.	* The tolerable range of the release rate is to be specified on pharmacokinetic and pharmacodynamic properties of the individual acitve ingredient.
* It is desirable that additional dissolution tests are conducted with the paddle method at 100 rpm at three pH levels (1.2; 4.0; 6.2), if an alternative method is to be used.	* If the correlation between the release rate and blood concentrations is not clear, it is desirable that the tolerable range be specified as within $\pm$5 % for the samples collected first, $\pm$10 % for collected next, and $\pm$15 % for those from the third collection.
* If there is some evidence that the release rate is accelerated by mechanical disintegrating effects, particularly preparations of an active ingredient with narrow therapeutic window may need to be additionally tested with mechanical disintegration (e.g. rotating flask method).	

Fig. 7: Guidelines for the Application for Product Approval of Oral Sustained Release Dosage Forms (Summary from ref. 3).

validity as a useful guide to the setting up of an in vitro-test programme for the characterization of the biopharmaceutical properties of controlled release preparations, e. g. within the context of independent comparative studies or in product development or for registration.

3. Validation of an in vitro-dissolution model

For a manufacturer to carry out his own quality control it is necessary to set up one individual in vitro-system for the routine testing for the release of batches of a certain product. For this the manufacturer could resort to a test model already used for extensive testing to assess the in vitro-dissolution properties (see above).

In each case it is necessary to validate the in vitro-dissolution model which entails providing proof that variations from the specified quality of the product being therapeutically relevant can be reliably recognized under the test conditions selected (discriminating potency). Conversely, there should be no significant differences between bioequivalent products in the in vitro-model.

True validation of an in vitro-dissolution model is therefore only possible by carrying out parallel in vivo- and in vitro-tests in order to present an in vivo/in vitro-association. However to confirm the suitability of the in vitro-test conditions employed it is not necessary to use a complicated mathematical correlation for the quantitative description of the plasma concentration-time-curve and the in vitro-dissolution function. A more pragmatic association, i. e. a linear relationship between a parameter that is relevant in vivo and one that is relevant in vitro, possibly also an identical ranking of different formulations in vivo and in vitro, should be regarded as adequate in this respect.

A proecedure of this type was also discussed at the Workshop on Controlled Release Dosage Forms (13). According to the appropriate recommendation for the development and validation of suitable in vitro-test conditions, the manufacture of at least three biopharmaceutically different formulations of the same controlled release principle is required. An in vitro-test should then be developped which will reveal the expected differences between the formulations in terms of the rate of dissolution of the active substance. The validation is carried out finally by investigating the absorption characteristics of the three formulations in a small group of subjects and comparing the pharmacokinetic data obtained with the results of in vitro-testing.

To confirm the suitability of an in vitro-test model that has been developped the comparative testing of preparations that are known to differ from the

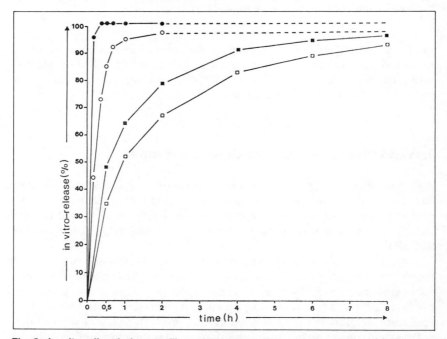

Fig. 8: In vitro-dissolution profiles of two immediate release (-●- capsules; -○- coated tablets) and two controlled release (-■-; -□-) Nifedipine products with different biopharmaceutical properties

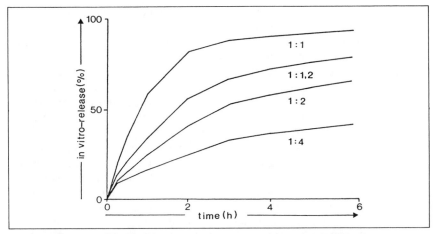

Fig. 9: Influence of coating thickness of microcapsules on their dissolution characteristics (ratio core: coating = 1:1; 1:1.2; 1:2; 1:4) (From Kaeser-Liard et al., ref. 14).

biopharmaceutical point of view can be evaluated without new in vivo-studies being to be performed. Thus to verify a model developped for the dissolution testing of nifedipine products two immediate release preparations which had been found in bioavailability studies to have differing plasma concentration-time-profiles were tested in vitro. In addition, two widely varying controlled-release nifedipine formulations were included in the tests. As can be seen from Fig. 8, the in vitro-model makes it possible to distinguish controlled-release from immediate release systems and portray biopharmaceutical differences within differing immediate release and controlled release preparations.

Proving plausibility of in vitro-test conditions for the formulation to be tested can if necessary be carried out without accompanying in vivo-tests or without knowing the results of bioavailability studies. Thus a test system can be shown to have adequate discriminating ability if, as is demonstrated in Fig. 9, differences in the degree of the extension of drug release to be expected in view of the galenical formulations are recognized as differences in the in vitro-rate of dissolution.

4. Specifications for in vitro-dissolution

Controlled release preparations are in principle required to release the active substance in a controlled, as far as possible quantitative manner within a reasonable period of time so that suitable plasma concentration-time-profiles are obtained. With active substances that are eliminated slowly (long elimination half-life) a more or less linear release will be advisable. With active substances that are eliminated rapidly an initial dose should be aimed for that will be more immediately released. Individual drug- and dosage form-specific properties should be taken into account for specification of dissolution profiles. However, to ensure that the drugs are safe and the controlled release preparations are of the quality that can be achieved with modern technology uniform dissolution characteristics from dosage form to dosage form (batch homogeneity) and uniform dissolution characteristics from production batch to production batch (batch conformity) should be required in any case.

The ideal case of dissolution of the active substance for a controlled release preparation is illustrated diagrammatically in Fig. 10. For the rate-determining control of the subsequent pharmacokinetic processes by the dissolution profile of the active substance it is necessary for the dissolution rate constant to be small in relation to the absorption rate constant. Moreover, in order to achieve adequate bioavailability the period of dissolution in vivo must be no longer than the dwell time of the controlled release dosage form in sections of the gastrointestinal tract that are capable of absorption. It should be noted that both, release rate konstant k_r and time period of drug release τ_r, are parameters of the in vivo-dissolution of the active substance which cannot always be extrapolated to the corresponding factors in vitro without transformation.

In order to lay down a theoretical profile for the dissolution of the active substance it is essential to understand the characteristic transport processes that take place during the passage through the gastrointestinal tract (Fig. 11). Thus information on the drug-specific absorption constant k_a which can

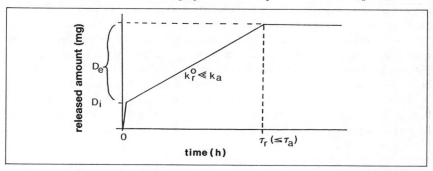

Fig. 10: Scheme of drug release from a controlled release dosage form (From Stricker, H., ref. 15)
D_i = initial dose
D_e = maintenance dose
k_a = rate constant of absorption
k_r = rate constant of drug release
τ_a = transit time of dosage from within absorption sites of the gastrointestinal tract
τ_r = time period of drug release

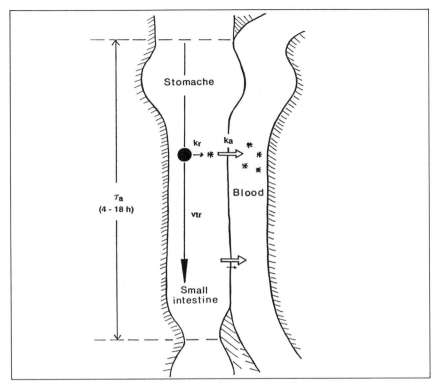

Fig 11: Scheme of transport processes during gastrointestinal transit (From Stricker, H., ref. 15)

k_a = rate constant of absorption
k_r = rate constant of drug release
V_{tr} = transport-rate of dosage form through the gastrointestinal tract
τ_a = transit time of dosage form within absorption sites of the gastrointestinal tract

assume differing proportions for different areas of the gastrointestinal tract is needed. The transport rate v_{tr} in the different sections of the gastrointestinal tract is basically determined by the dosage form. With a number of dosage forms gastric emptying can for example represent the rate-determining step for the in vitro-dissolution of the active substance. Moreover with monolith dosage forms v_{tr} is exposed to greater variability than with multiple unit forms, e. g. pellets. Finally, the time-dependent absorption kinetics (k_a) and the longitudinal gastrointestinal transport kinetics (v_{tr}) jointly determine the dwell time τ_a in sections of the gastrointestinal tract that are capable of absorption.

The requirement profile for the dissolution of the active substance of controlled release preparations can therefore only be individually compiled with the knowledge of the pharmacokinetic properties of the drug in question and the transport properties of the dosage form selected. Moreover, pharmacodynamic factors, especially the therapeutic range, are important when stipulating the tolerance limits to be accepted in quality control and for the total shelf-life of the preparation once the theoretical curve ist established.

As the standardization of in vitro-test conditions for controlled-release preparations has been already assessed as extremely problematic, it is virtually impossible to standardize the requirement profiles for the dissolution of the active substance of controlled release drugs. The USP Policy on Modified-release Dosage Forms must be criticized in this respect (see Fig. 6). Although in the description of the requirement profile as a function of the dosage interval, the test can be seen indirectly to take account of kinetic processes, it does not ensure that proper and scientifically adequate consideration is given to the pharmacokinetic properties. It is especially unacceptable to establish the tolerance limits irrespective of the pharmacodynamic profile of the active substance in question. In this respect the introductory comments on the USP Policy are possibly understandable and consequently it is expected that the majority of controlled release preparations to be described will not be classified in the category given under case 1.

A basic prerequisite for establishing a requirement profile for the in vitro-dissolution of controlled release preparations as a function of the dosage interval is a correlation or at least a linear relationship between the temporal course of the in vitro- and in vivo-dissolution. This accounts not only for the

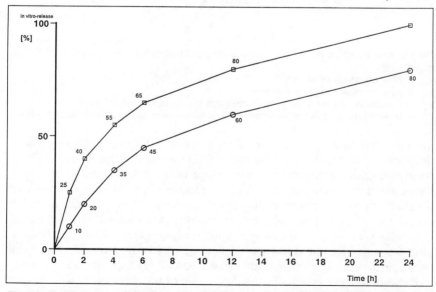

Fig. 12: Drug release requirements for Indomethacin Extended-Release Capsules for a dosage interval of 12 hours (From ref. 16)

criticism of the USP Policy on Modified-release Dosage Forms but also for the need for a critical examination of the appropriate monographs or monograph proposals for controlled-release preparations. Thus for (Fig. 12) Indomethacin Extended Release Capsules (16), assuming a dosage interval of twelve hours, a release of at least 80% of the declared amount is required within 24 hours. Tests have shown however that indomethacin is sufficiently rapidly and completely absorbed form controlled release capsules during the usual passage through the gastrointestinal tract over a period of only five hours (17).

A more sensible approach to the standardization of the specifications for the in vitro-dissolution testing for controlled release preparations is adopted in the Japanese registration guidelines (Fig. 7) which state that the theoretical profile for the dissolution of the active substance can only be individually established by taking account of the pharmacokinetic properties. The standardization proposal laid down in the Japanese guidelines then covers the selection of the measuring intervals for in vitro-dissolution and an attempt for the specification of tolerance limits.

Extensive experience of the association of in vitro-dissolution results with pharmacokinetic data from corresponding in vivo-studies is essential for the elaboration and validation of useful in vitro-test models and for laying down relevant requirement profiles and tolerance limits, as is so neatly summed up and required in the report on the Workshop on Controlled Release Dosage Forms (13): 'It is generally accepted by pharmaceutical scientists that the present state of science and technology does not permit consistently meaningful in vitro versus in vivo-correlations for extended release dosage forms. Development of such methodology remains a future objective'.

5. Literature

(1) Joint Report of the Section for Control Laboratories and the Section of Industrial Pharmacists of the FIP: Guidelines for Dissolution Testing of Solid Oral Products. Pharm. Ind. *43*, 334–343 (1981)

(2) USP Policy on Modified-release Dosage Forms: Pharm. Forum *9*, 2999–3001 (1983)

(3) Guidelines for the Application for Product Approval of Oral Sustained Release Dosage Forms Ministry of Health and Welfare, Japan, 1987

(4) Bundesvereinigung Deutscher Apothekerverbände – ABDA (Ed.) Deutscher Arzneimittel-Codex. Govi-Verlag GmbH, Pharmazeutischer Verlag, Frankfurt, 1986

(5) Möller, H.: Biopharmaceutical Assessment of Modified Release Oral Dosage Forms, Pharm. Ind. *48*, 514–519 (1986)

(6) Graepel, P. H., Momberger, H., Kuhn, D.: BIO-DIS – Ein Gerät zur Prüfung der in vitro-Freisetzung von Retardarzneimitteln. Pharm. Ztg. *131*, 1820–1823 (1986)

(7) Ostrowski, J., Voegele, D., Brockmeier, D., von Hattingberg, H. M., Blasini, R., Bruegmann, U., Resag, K., Rudolph, W., Weidemann, H. In vivo-Relevanz von in vitro-Liberationsergebnissen. Acta Pharm. Technol. *29*, 295–301 (1983)

(8) Koch, H. P.: The Rotating Flask Method. Pharm. Ind. *44*, 838–842 (1982)

(9) Winde, E.: Erfahrungen mit der rotierenden Durchflußzelle (RD-Zelle). Acta Pharm. Technol. *26*, 180–195 (1980)

(10) Herzfeldt, D. C., Lambov, N.: Untersuchungen zur in vitro/in vivo-Korrelation der Absorptionskinetik von Indometacin mit

einem Durchflußlösemodell. Acta Pharm. Technol. *32,* 43–48 (1986)

(11) Skelly, J. P., Yan, M. K., Elkins, J. S., Yamamoto, L. A., Shah, V. P., Barr, W. H.: Drug. Devel. and Indus. Pharmacy 12, 1177–1201 (1986)

(12) Verhoeven, J., Peschier, L. J. C., Danhof, M., Junginger, H. E.: Optimization of Oral Dosage Form Design: A new in vitro Food-Interaction Model. Paper given at the Third European Congress on Biopharmaceutics and Pharmacokinetics, Freiburg, 1985

(13) Report of the Workshop on Controlled Release Dosage Forms: Issues and Controversies, Cosponsored by Food and Drug Administration, Academy of Pharmaceutical Science, and American Association for Clinical Pharmacology & Therapeutics, Washington, D.C. (1985)

(14) Kaeser-Liard, B., Kissel, T., Sucker, H.: Manufacture of Controlled Release Formulations by a new Microencapsulation Process, the Emulsion-Induction Technique. Acta Pharm. Technol. *30,* 249–301 (1984)

(15) Stricker, H.: Biopharmazeutische Beurteilung von peroralen Retardzubereitungen. Paper given at the International APV Symposium Bioavailability/Bioequivalence, Pharmaceutical and Therapeutic Equivalence in Würzburg from 9–11 Feb. 1987

(16) Pharm. Forum (1987) 13: 2618

(17) Möller, H.: Chapter IV.

IX. Associations Between In Vitro and In Vivo

Martin Nicklasson, Södertälje, Sweden

Summary

In vitro dissolution testing is an important corner-stone in the biopharmaceutical science for a successful drug delivery research. Thus far, many attempts have been described in the literature in order to establish various kinds of associations or correlations between in vitro-dissolution and some in vivo-parameters. By applying mathematical principles such as linear system analysis or moment analysis, analogous data describing in vitro as well as in vivo-processes can be obtained which opens new dimensions for the formulator to interpret the dosage form behaviour. It may also be possible to define critical parameters in terms of biopharmaceutical properties of the product.

This presentation will show and discuss important aspects on in vitro dissolution testing and its association to in vivo in order to scrutinize a solid dosage form during the development phases. Different association methods will be discussed, and in some cases, the limitations with such methods will be emphasized.

The main objectives with in vitro-dissolution testing is to serve as a guidance to the formulator regarding product design and in quality control. Even if in vitro-dissolution testing cannot replace in vivo bioavailability assessment, it can still give valuable biopharmaceutical information. When absorption data are available, possibilities arise to establish associations to in vivo. If mathematical principles such as linear system analysis are applied, new and interesting dimensions may be generated for making advanced desicions in the formulation work. It is the aim with this presentation to examplify methods for in vitro dissolution testing and the possibility of establishing associations to in vivo in a routine development work on solid dosage forms.

1. In Vitro dissolution testing

The well acknowledged compendial methods for in vitro-dissolution testing such as the paddle and basket methods can be regarded as closed system stirring methods which operates under finite sink conditions. This paper will not reveal further details about these methods since they are already known to

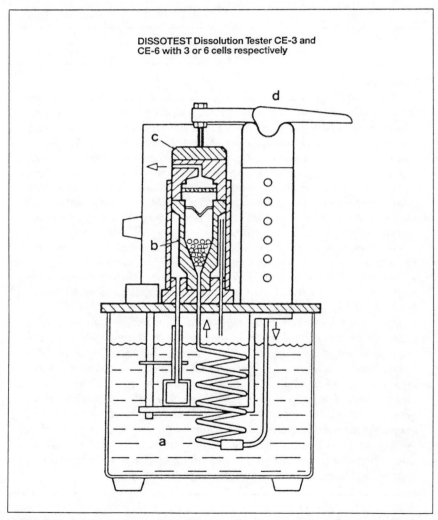

Fig. 1: Schematic presentation of the flow through dissolution apparatus. Cross section: a) warming bath b) 'flow through cell' c) filter head d) clamping device.

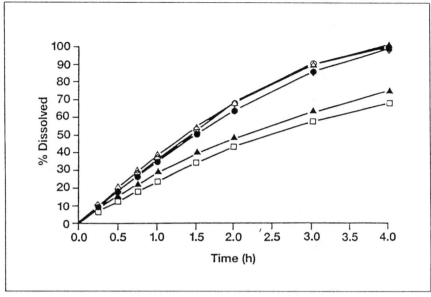

Fig. 2: Percent salicylic acid dissolved vs time at pH 7.4 using the flow through method at 16 ml/min. Mean curves, USP calibrator tablets Lot H; ○ Laboratory 1, ● Laboratory 2, ◇ Laboratory 3, △ Laboratory 4, ▲ Laboratory 4 without deaerated medium, □ Laboratory 5 without deaerated medium.

the man skilled in the art. However, one can easily define the limitations of these methods, e.g. for poorly soluble compounds, particularly small multiparticulate systems which may adhere to the analytical devices, floating systems etc.

Another approach would be to operate under infinite sink conditions by applying an open flow through method. Several papers have been published showing the application of the flow through method on solid dosage forms (1–3). In a recent paper, a collaborative study was performed among several independent laboratories showing that the flow through method can generate reproducible data in comparison with the compendial paddle method (4). Fig. 1 shows a schematic drawing of the flow through apparatus.

The dosage form is placed in the flow through cell and the dissolution medium is then pumped through the cell hence achieving an infinite sink condition. In Fig. 2, the mean in vitro-dissolution curves for the USP salicylic acid calibrator tablets are shown obtained in the collaborative study mentioned above. The data reveal the importance of using well defined dissolution medium in terms of deaeration, otherwise a misleading picture of the release rate will be obtained. The laboratories which first generated the two lower curves, repeated the test after an adequate pretreatment of the dissolution

	Flow-through method			USP XXI Paddle method	
	8 ml/min	16 ml/min	50 ml/min	50 rpm	100 rpm
20%					
Lab 1	5	3	–	13	8
Lab 2	11	4	4	12	4
Lab 3	12	8	1	9	6
Lab 4	31	5	5	13	4
40%					
Lab 1	2	2	–	13	7
Lab 2	6	4	3	12	4
Lab 3	9	4	1	8	6
Lab 4	3	1	4	11	3
80%					
Lab 1	3	1	–	9	4
Lab 2	3	4	2	7	3
Lab 3	6	2	2	8	6
Lab 4	–	1	5	7	4

**Fig. 3: Coefficient of variation (n=6) for the time to dissolve 20, 50 and 80 % of sali-
cylic acid obtained by each laboratory using either the flow through method or the
USP XXI paddle method.**

medium and the data thus obtained were found to be in accordance with the
data found for the other collaborative laboratories. The overall variations
obtained in the collaborative study are summarized in Fig. 3.

As can be seen, the flow through method was capable of generating uniform
data with small variations within and among the different laboratories compared to the USP paddle method.

Dissolution experiments conducted with different methods may help to
explain why a given dosage form behaves in a certain way after administration
in vivo. In order to increase the fundamental understanding in terms of in
vitro-dissolution properties for a dosage form and to find a discriminating
quality control method, various hydrodynamic principles should be investigated. If results can be generated by various methods, the most pertinent test
conditions can be selected for future quality control. Some studies have shown
that the USP paddle method are advantageous whereas other reports reveal
the importance of using the flow through method. Not only should different in
vitro-methods be studied for a new drug formulation but also various experimental conditions within each method. In Fig. 4, the in vitro-dissolution is
shown for remoxipride controlled release pellets determined in different dissolution media. The data shown in Fig 4 for remoxipride do not indicate any

serious problems regarding the choice of dissolution method or test condition.

Fig. 5 however, shows the in vitro-dissolution profiles for a controlled release tablet of a new CNS compound using the USP paddle method at different static pH conditions. As can be seen, the dissolution rate decreases substantially at higher pH. These kind of test conditions cannot be regarded as physiologically relevant, since the pH changes from low values into higher ones as the drug formulation passas through the gastrointestinal tract.

The in vitro-dissolution testing was therefore conducted using the flow through method, and during the test, the pH was changed as a function of time. Fig. 6 shows the in vitro-dissolution curve generated by applying this methodology and, as can be seen, a complete in vitro-dissolution was obtained after about 12 hours even if higher pH values were applied in late phases of the test. This indicates that there may be no limitations regarding drug absorption in vivo due to incomplete drug release from the dosage form. This was also confirmed in a bioavailability study showing that the new CNS compound was readily absorbed when formulated as a controlled release tablet having an in vitro-release pattern as shown in Fig. 6.

Thus, by applying different test methods and test conditions in a drug

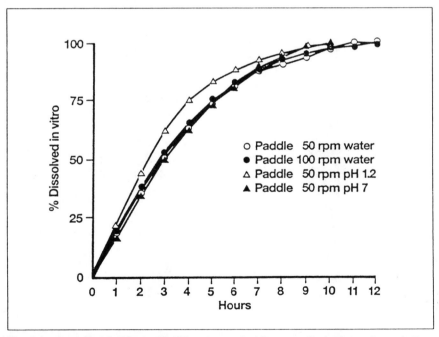

Fig. 4: In vitro-dissolution profiles for a remoxipride controlled release formulation using various experimental conditions for the paddle method.

design program, a solid ground will be created for a fundamental understanding about the properties of the product which may be used in future associations to in vivo.

2. In vitro/in vivo associations

Associations between in vitro and in vivo using empirical single value parameters or nonanalogous data have been commonly applied in the past. This approach has in many cases been shown to be sufficient for obtaining some

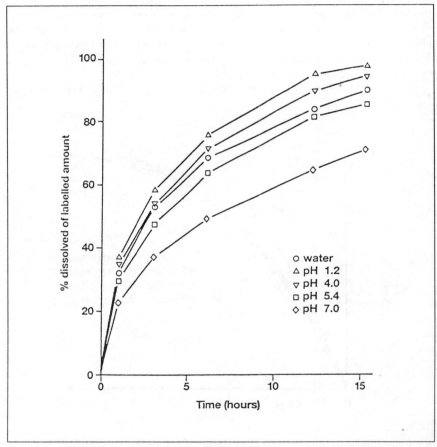

Fig. 5: In vitro-dissolution of a new anxiolytic compound in a controlled release tablet using the USP XXI paddle at 50 rpm.

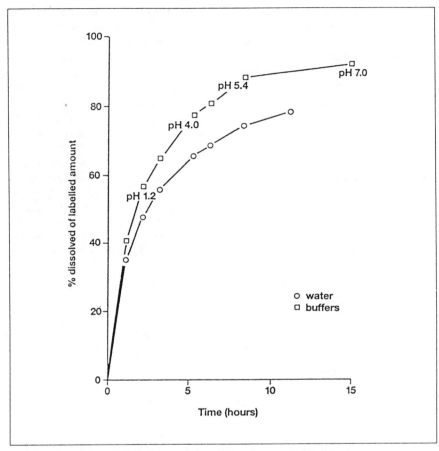

Fig. 6: In vitro-dissolution of a new anxiolytic compound formulated in a controlled release tablet using the flow through method at 16 ml/min.

kind of relationship between in vitro and in vivo and this concept is still common in the biopharmaceutical literature. By the introduction of moment analysis and linear system analysis, the possibility to associate analogous data in a quantitative way has become a reality. The mean residence time of a drug molecule following administration in a given dosage form can easily be calculated from the ratio between the area under the first moment of the plasma concentration versus time curve and the area under the zero moment of the same curve as show by Eq. (1).

$$\text{MRT} = \frac{\int_0^\infty t \cdot C \, dt}{\int_0^\infty C \, dt} \qquad (1)$$

The mean residence time constitutes several kinetic processes and can thus be rather complex in nature. By treating the in vitro-dissolution data in the same way, i.e. taking the ratio between the area under the first moment of the in vitro-dissolution rate curve and the area under the zero moment of the same curve, a corresponding expression for time is obtained. However, this time expression is denoted the mean in vitro-dissolution time. By plotting the mean residence time versus the mean in vitro-dissolution time it is now possible to associate in vitro with in vivo using data generated by means of the same mathematical principle as can be seen in Fig. 7 which shows data for alaproclate administered in different controlled release dosage forms.

In Fig. 7, the intercept, i.e. where the mean in vitro-dissolution time is equal to zero, is close to the calculated mean residence time obtained for an oral aqueous solution of the corresponding drug compound, which hence support the validity of the association. If the in vivo study also includes an aqueous solution of the drug, it is possible to calculate the mean in vitro-dissolution time by deducting the mean residence time for the oral solution from the mean residence time obtained for the solid test formulation. Fig. 8

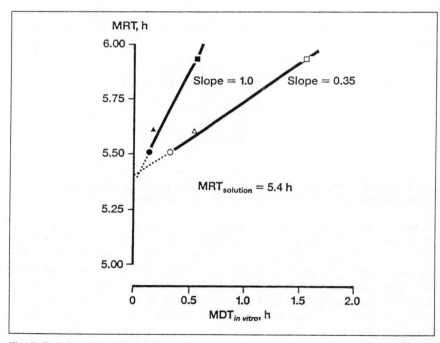

Fig. 7: Relationship between mean residence time, MRT, and mean dissolution time in vitro, MDT, for conventional alaproclate tablets 100 mg. Closed symbols = Paddle method 100 rpm, pH 1.2, open symbols = Paddle method 50 rpm, pH 1.2.

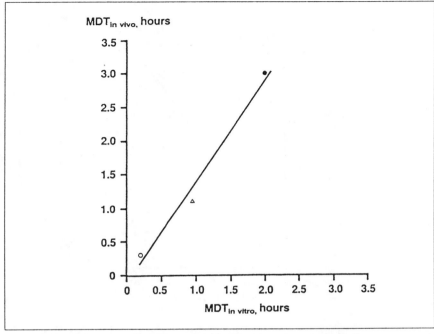

Fig. 8: Relationship between mean dissolution time, MDT, in vitro and mean dissolution time in vivo for different conventional remoxipride tablets 10 mg. ○ **formulation A,** △ **formulation B,** ● **formulation C.**

shows an example where the mean in vivo-dissolution time has been plotted versus the mean in vitro-dissolution time for different remoxipride tablets. As can be seen, a good association has been established and the slope indicates that the association is a sensitive model for future in vivo predictions when using mean in vitro-dissolution time data.

For this kind of relationship, the intercept should be equal to zero which is nearly the case in Fig. 8. What more information can be obtained from such relationships than a demonstration of a general in vitro in vivo correlation? Fig. 9 shows the consequences of plotting the mean in vitro-dissolution time versus the mean in vivo-dissolution time for different alaproclate tablets using two different agitation conditions for the paddle method in vitro.

Both agitation conditions (50 and 100 rpm) at pH 1.2 show excellent correlations to in vivo but, as can be seen, the slopes differ significantly. The slope at 100 rpm was found to be about 0.9 whereas the slope at 50 rpm was found to be only 0.3. It seems as if the 100 rpm condition is a more sensitive test condition for this particularly drug product due to the steeper slope in the association plot. Also, the fact that a slope close to unity has been obtained

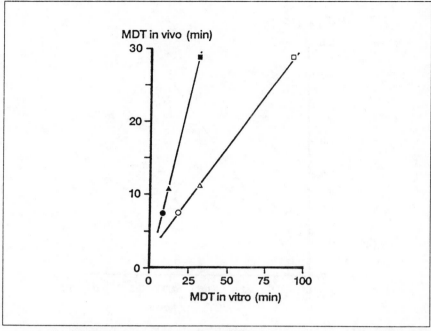

Fig. 9: Relationship between mean dissolution time in vitro and mean dissolution time in vivo (MDT) for different alaproclate tablets 100 mg using different agitation conditions in vitro (Paddle method pH 1.2). Closed symbols = 100 rpm, slope = 0.85, open symbols = 50 rpm, slope = 0.28.

gives further support for using this test condition in future tests on alaproclate tablets. By correlating analogous data in this way, the formulator will be able to select the most pertinent in vitro test conditions to be used in the development work or in quality control of the product.

The value of the zero moment, i. e. the area under the plasma concentration versus time curve, can also be used when associating in vitro and in vivo moments. An example is given in Fig. 10 for a penicillin derivative demonstrating a drug system where the extent of bioavailability seems to be relatively sensitive for changes in drug dissolution time.

In vitro in vivo associations regarding drug dissolution can also be made in a quantitative way by means of linear system analysis, applying the principle of deconvolution. It is thus possible to compare the entire in vitro-dissolution process with the same process in vivo. This can be seen in Fig. 11 where individual in vivo dissolution profiles obtained in six healthy volunteers for a remoxipride controlled release formulation are compared with the in vitro dissolution process obtained by using the flow through method in water. These

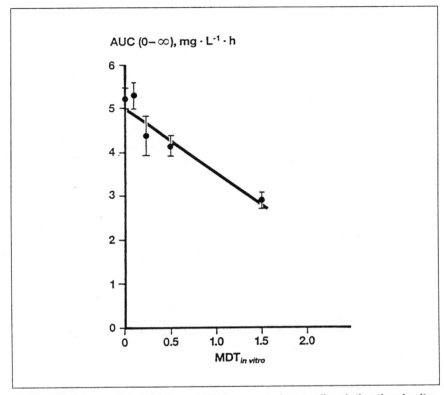

Fig. 10: Association between mean AUC ± s.e.m. and mean dissolution time in vitro (MDT) for different microcapsule formulations of a penicillin derivative administered to healthy volunteers, n=12. USP XXI paddle method 100 rpm, pH 1.2.

associations make it possible, on an intraindividual basis, to evaluate when in time a correspondence exists and when in time any deviation may occur between in vitro- and in vivo-dissolution.

An important criterion to consider in a drug development program is the impact of various formulation factors on the biopharmaceutical properties of the formulation. By means of convolution, the opposite process of deconvolution, it is possible to predict or construct hypothetical plasma concentration versus time courses based upon in vitro dissolution data. The only thing necessary, besides the in vitro-dissolution data, is a weighting function, i. e. plasma concentration data after administration of an oral aqueous solution of the drug. If these criteria are fulfilled, important biopharmaceutical desicions can be made in direct connection with the practical formulation work which indeed creates new dimensions for an optimal drug design. However, the association model applied must be validated for a given drug compound

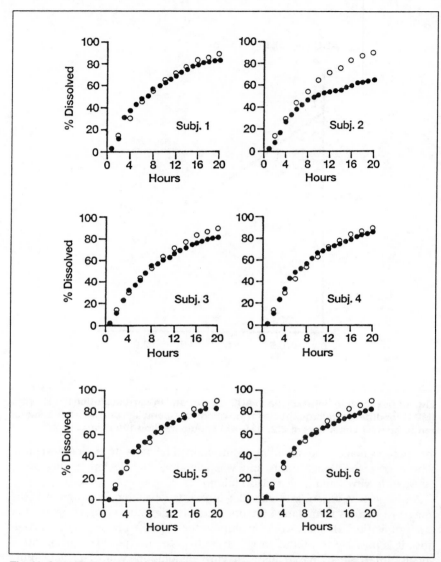

Fig. 11: Associations between in vitro-dissolution (○) and in vivo dissolution obtained by means of numerical deconvolution (●) for remoxipride controlled release microcapsules 100 mg. In vitro = flow through apparatus, water, 16 ml/min.

before it can be used in a routine work. Fig. 12 shows observed and predicted plasma concentration versus time courses for remoxipride tablets with different in vitro-dissolution properties. It is quite obvious from the results in Fig. 12 that numerical convolution is a useful instrument for predicting an in vivo response for remoxipride due to changes in in vitro-dissolution rate and that the predicted values closely correspond to the actual situation.

3. Limitations for in vitro/in vivo associations

The data presented thus far have been quite ideal and, nice associations between in vitro and in vivo have been shown. However, the in vitro-dissolution test methods mentioned previously may not be applicable or, pharmacokinetic or physiological problems may exist which can cause difficulties regarding in vitro in vivo associations. Before applying various in vitro in vivo association methods, a fundamental understanding about the physicochemical

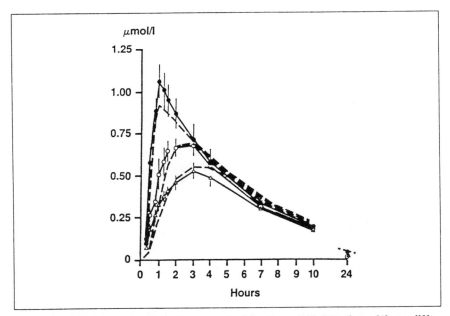

Fig. 12: Plasma concentrations for remoxipride after administration of three different tablet formulations 20 mg in ten healthy volunteers. Mean values ± s.e.m.; ● formulation A, ○ formulation B, △ formulation C. Dotted lines denote the predicted plasma concentrations obtained by means of numerical convolution, $\Delta t = 0.25$ h.

as well as the pharmacokinetic properties of the drug compound must exist. For drugs with extremely low aqueous solubility, pH dependent dissolution, absorption rate limited bioavailability, site specific absorption, first pass metabolism, hydrolytic or enzymatic degradation in the gastrointestinal tract etc., problems may arise. Fig. 13 shows an attempt to calculate a hypothetical plasma concentration versus time course by means of numerical convolution for a new CNS compound.

As can be seen, there is a large deviation between the predicted and observed time courses which cannot be explained by an inadequate in vitro-dissolution testing. This particulary drug compound shows an extremely high

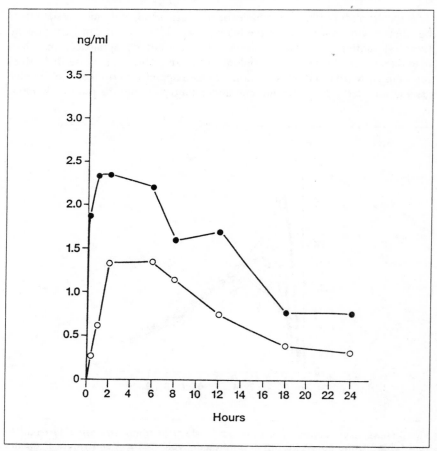

Fig. 13: Observed (●) and predicted (○) plasma concentration versus time courses for a new CNS compound formulated in a controlled release tablet. Mean values. The predicted time course was generated by means of numerical convolution.

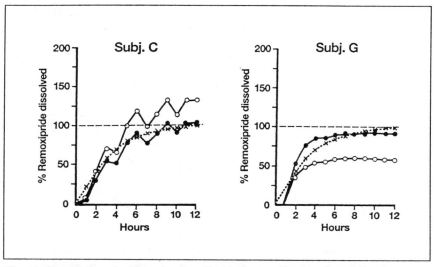

Fig. 14: Associations between in vitro-dissolution and in vivo-dissolution for remoxipride controlled release microcapsules in two healthy volunteers. (... x ... x ..) in vitro, flow through method, water, 16 ml/min, (O) in vivo by means of numerical deconvolution, (●) in vivo by means of numerical deconvolution considering equal availability of the test and reference formulations in the gastrintestinal tract (From Nicklasson, M. et al., ref. 5).

first pass metabolism and hence this phenomenon disqualifies the drug for use in a linear system analysis. However, even if a drug is used which does not show any of the above mentioned limitations, there is still a risk of obtaining a misleading picture of the actual amount of drug dissolved in vivo when applying moment or linear system analysis due to intraindividual variations in the absorption process from one administration to another. A paper has recently suggested a way of calculating the cumulative amount of drug dissolved in vivo when numerical deconvolution is applied assuming equal availability of the test and reference formulations in the gastrointestinal tract (5). Fig. 14 shows the calculated amount of remoxipride dissolved from a controlled release formulation in vivo by means of deconvolution in two healthy subjects compared with the in vitro-dissolution profile obtained with the flow through method at 16 ml/min in water.

The open circles show the result when deconvolution was applied on the plasma raw data without considering the actual extent of bioavailability obtained after administration, on two separate occasions, of the test and reference formulations respectively. The solid circles show the same in vivo-dissolution process if this was done. As can be seen from the solid circles, more precise associations are obtained in both subjects if the extent of drug absorption of the test and reference formulations is considered in the calculations. If this is not done, absurd values may be generated as can be seen for subject C showing a value of 140% dissolvend in vivo.

Fig. 15 shows rather poor associations between in vitro- and in vivo-dissolution for a penicillin derivative using water as dissolution medium.

However, a pH dependent in vitro-dissolution was found for this drug

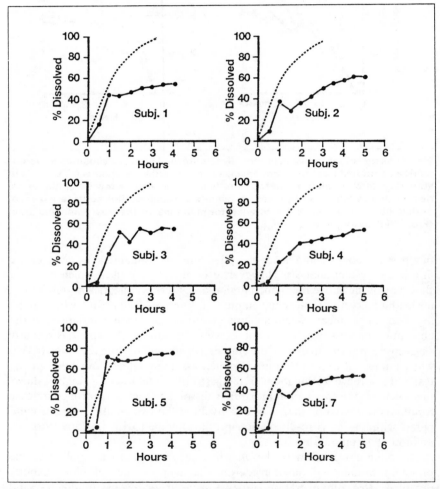

Fig. 15: Associations between in vitro-dissolution and in vivo-dissolution in six healthy volunteers for a microcapsule formulations of a penicillin derivative. (.......) in vitro-dissolution, flow through method, water, 16 ml/min, (●) in vivo-dissolution calculated by means of numerical deconvolution, $\triangle t = 0.5$ h.

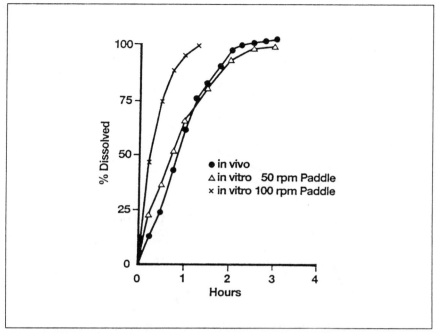

Fig. 16: Associations between in vitro-dissolution and in vivo-dissolution for an Ala-proclate tablet formulation 200 mg. The in vivo-dissolution profile was obtained by using numerical deconvolution.

formulation showing a much slower in vitro dissolution at low pH values. Hence, a better but not ideal picture was found if in vitro-dissolution data obtained at pH 1.2 were used instead. The pH dependent in vitro-dissolution process is probably not the only explanation why a relatively poor in vitro in vivo association was obtained for this formulation. It is well known that penicillins exhibit a limited absorption capacity in the distal parts of the gastrointestinal tract which also may contribute in explaining the phenomenon shown in Fig. 15. Not only pH but also inadequate hydrodynamic conditions may cause difficulties when one is trying to create an in vitro in vivo association. This was demonstrated previously for moment analysis. The results in Fig. 16 for alaproclate tablets applying deconvolution and the USP paddle method at pH 1.2 demonstrate the necessity of selecting relevant agitation conditions in order to be able to generate a proper in vitro in vivo association. Obviously, 50 rpm corresponds best to the in vivo situation for this formulation.

In vitro-dissolution methods have been described for explaining the effect of fat food on the release and absorption of drugs, e. g. for theophylline, from

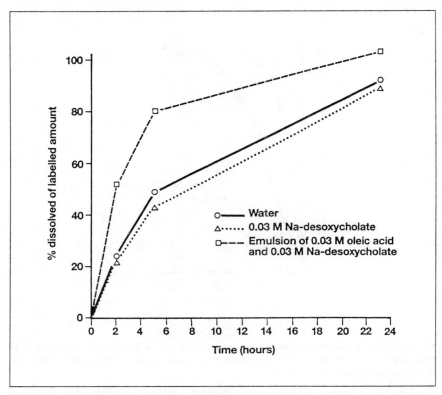

Fig. 17: In vitro-dissolution of a benzamide microcapsule formulation in three different dissolution media using the USP XXI paddle method at 100 rpm.

controlled release products. The products were soaked in oleic acid for 1 to 3 hours prior to dissolution testing. The influence of fat can also be studied in vitro by exposing the formulation to an oil in water emulsion. Fig. 17 shows the in vitro-dissolution profiles for a benzamide multiparticulate controlled release formulation in an emulsion of sodium desoxycholate and oleic acid in water, compared to the same process obtained in water with and without the surfactant, using the USP paddle method at 100 rpm.

As can be seen, a far more rapid in vitro-dissolution was found in the lipid emulsion than in the aqueous media. If the same formulation was first soaked in oleic acid for 3 hours, as mentioned previously, and then tested for in vitro dissolution, about 98% of the drug content was found to be released within 2 hours. Based on these results, one might suspect a great impact on drug release and drug absorption when this formulation is to be taken together with a fat meal. However, this was not found when tested in healthy subjects. The average AUC values were found to be decreased by about 20% when fat food was taken together with the formulation compared to the fasting condition. Obviously, the in vitro model used does not reflect the in vivo situation in an adequate way. The solubility parameters for oleic acid and the film forming agent for the controlled release membrane (ethyl cellulose) were interestingly found to be almost identical. Thus, oleic acid is a perfect solvent for ethyl cellulose. This simple situation will not exist in vivo since many other factors may influence the drug release and drug absorption when the formulation is taken together with a fat meal.

4. Conclusion

Before the application of various in vitro in vivo association methods, a fundamental understanding about the physicochemical properties as well as the pharmacokinetic and absorption properties of the drug compound must exist. For drugs showing an extremely low aqueous solubility, pH dependent dissolution, absorption rate limited bioavailability, site specific absorption, high first pass metabolism, hydrolytic/enzymatic degradation in the GI tract, problems may occur. It is therefore of outmost importance that a careful validation of the association modell is conducted otherwise erroneous conclusions may be drawn. However, if a validated association model has been established, a powerful biopharmaceutical tool will be available for a successful drug design work.

5. Literature

(1) Langenbucher, F.: In vitro assessment of dissolution kinetics: Description and evaluation of a column-type method. J. Pharm. Sci. *58*, 1265–1272 (1969)

(2) Möller, H.: Dissolution testing of different dosage forms using the flow through method. Pharm. Ind. *45*, 617–622 (1983)

(3) Möller, H.: Biopharmaceutical assessment of modified release oral dosage forms. Proceedings from the 45th International Congress of Pharmaceutical Sciences, September 1985, F.I.P., Montreal

(4) Nicklasson, M., Wennergren, B., Lindberg, J., Persson, C., Ahlgren, R., Palm, B., Pettersson, A., Wenngren, L.: A collaborative in vitro dissolution study using the flow through method. Int. J. Pharm. *37*, 195–202 (1987)

(5) Nicklasson, M., Graffner, C., Nilsson, M.-I.: Assessment of in vivo drug dissolution by means of numerical deconvolution considering gastrointestinal availability. Int. J. Pharm. *40*, 165–171 (1987)

X. Regulatory Recommendations in USA on Investigation and Evaluation of Oral Controlled Release Products

J. Skelly, Rockville

SUMMARY

Differences in the terminology used by FDA and USP are addressed as are various rationale for making and dosing controlled release dosage forms. Criteria for substituting pharmacokinetic studies in lieu of clinical studies are elucidated. The relationship between pharmacodynamics, pharmacokinetics, and in vitro data has been explored and the basic drug application requirements explained. Functional tolerance, fluctuation, site specific absorption, first pass metabolism, dose dumping, food effect, diurinal variation and their importance to the approval process are discussed as are the types of pharmacokinetic and biopharmaceutic studies that need to be conducted. Requirement differences for non-oral dosage forms are explained.

1. General Considerations

As the FDA is charged with establishing the safety and effectiveness of new drug products, approval of New Drug Applications for a new chemical entity, initially marketed in Controlled Release Dosage Forms, must have clinical studies in patients to establish its safety and efficacy. It is necessary under the safety provisions to determine the bioavailability of each new dosage form. The pharmacokinetics which describe the absorption, distribution, metabolism and elimination of each chemical entity in a dosage form and justification of the dosage regimen recommended in the labelling need to be submitted.

Controlled release dosage forms are defined by the F.D.A. as those formulations designed to release an active ingredient(s), at rates which differ significantly from their corresponding immediate release forms. Many terms have been used to describe these forms, e. g., delayed action, extended action, gradual release, prolonged release, protracted release, repeat action, slow release, sustained release, depot, retard, and timed release dosage forms. Any of these terms, or similar terms which impart the same idea, may be used in labelling to designate a controlled release product. The Agency generally uses the following terminology:

A. **Oral Dosage**
  1. Delayed Release Drug Products
  2. Prolonged Release Drug Products
B. **Intramuscular Dosage**
  1. Depot Injections
  2. Water Immiscible Injections, i. e., oils
C. **Cutaneous/Subcutaneous Dosage**
  1. Implants
  2. Transdermal Preparations
D. **Targeted Dosage Form**
  1. Ocusert
  2. IUD's
  3. Pumps

The type of controlled release product to be developed is often determined by the physicochemical, pharmacokinetic, and/or pharmacological properties of a drug. In some instances, products may have characteristics of more than a single type.

In the case of delayed release products the primary objective is to target drug release at a specific time and/or site. The best examples are enteric coated products, whose purpose would be to prevent drug release in the acid environment of the stomach because of possible drug degradation or stomach irritation, yet enable drug release in the more alkaline environment of the intestinal tract, at a site high enough so as to still permit sufficient time for full drug absorption.

Prolonged release drug products are often formulated to permit the establishment and maintenance of drug and/or metabolite(s) concentration at sites for longer intervals of time than is possible with conventional drugs, so as to provide a clinical advantage. An example would be Theophylline controlled release.

The term 'Long acting' has been used for those drug substances which have an inherently long pharmacological effect, because of their physical chemical properties (for example – drugs having a half-life greater than 12 hours). In general, controlled release oral dosage forms of drugs with long half-lives have been judged by the Agency as not having sufficient rationale, in as much as they generally produce little change in the glood concentration after multiple doses have been administered. On the other hand, the existence of such products have been justified on the basis of their ability to minimize toxicity and the occurrence of adverse reactions, as well as on the basis of providing greater patient convenience and better patient compliance. Our terminology also recognizes intramuscular injections, implants, cutaneous and targeted dosage forms.

The oral controlled release drug product classes have been referred to by the U.S.P. as "Modified Release." Although the F.D.A. regulations specify "Controlled Release", they include more than oral controlled release products.

2. Rationale

The obvious advantage of controlled release drug delivery is the increase in the time interval required between doses. This provides for a decrease in the number of doses per day. Additionally, controlled release dosage should be accompanied by a reduction in the fluctuation of drug blood levels about the mean, by decreasing C_{max} and increasing C_{min}, for drugs with a narrow therapeutic index. This may be accompanied by decrease in toxicity, or if a threshold concentration is required, increase in efficacy. The degree of fluctu-

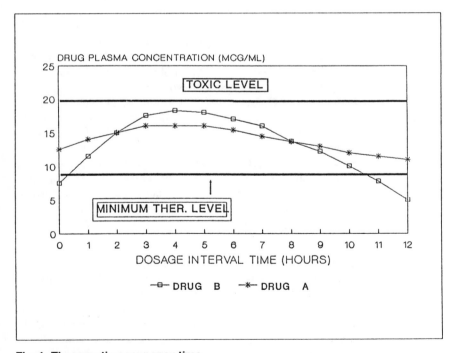

Fig. 1: Therapeutic occupancy time

ation about the mean plasma level is therefore an important parameter for regulatory assessment. A second criterion is the time that the plasma concentration stays within therapeutic range "therapeutic occupancy time". (Fig. 1).

3. Regulatory requirements

Approval of such a drug delivery system requires submission of data to substantiate the clinical safety and efficacy (if not otherwise known), of the product and demonstration of its controlled drug release characteristics. Controlled clinical studies may be required to demonstrate the safety and efficacy of the drug(s) depending upon what is known about the drug substance. Additionally, drug bioavailability data on the controlled release formulation is required. Such data may be acceptable in lieu of clinical trials.

The extent to which these potential advantages are realized must be evaluated for each specific drug entity especially with respect to he therapeutic window. Since many biological systems are complex homeostatic systems with a variety of feedback loops, which exhibit cyclical or diurnal behaviour, one cannot assume that the ideal plasma level is a constant steady state. Data obtained from studies on transdermal patches strongly suggest that the non varying plasma levels of nitroglycerin results in the development of tolerance. The fundamental question then in developing a controlled release product of an already approved immediate release dosage form is, whether clinical safety and efficacy data will be required, or whether a pharmacokinetics evaluation will suffice. The question was addressed at workshop sponsored by FDA, AAPS, ASCPT and DIA in October 1985 (1), it concluded that:

A rational answer to that question must be based upon an evaluation of the available data of the drug's pharmacodynamics, as well as its pharmacokinetics. Where there is a well defined relationship between plasma concentration of drug and/or active metabolite(s) and clinical response (therapeutic and adverse), it may be possible to rely on plasma concentration data alone as a basis for approval of the controlled release product. This is particularly so when the degree of fluctuation

$$\frac{C_{max} - C_{min}}{C_{av}}$$

for the release product administered is already small.

Where the therapeutic effect is indirect, where irreversible toxicity can occur, where there is evidence of functional (pharmacodynamic) tolerance, where peak to trough differences of the immediate release product are very large, or where there is any other reasonable uncertainty concerning the relationship between plasma concentration and therapeutic and adverse effects, it will probably be necessary to a carry out clinical studies.

Where there is no well defined relationship between the pharmacokinetics and pharmacodynamics of a drug, the premarketing evaluation of the controlled release product should include consideration of the possible development of functional tolerance to the drug. The premarketing evaluation should also include consideration of the possible occurrence of sensitivity reactions or local tissue damage due to dosage form dependent persistence or localization of the drug, the clinical implications of dose dumping, or unexpected decrease of bioavailability (by physiological or physicochemical mechanisms), and quantitative alteration in the metabolic fate of the drug due to nonlinear or site specific disposition.

The elucidation of the therapeutic, pharmacodynamic pharmacokinetic and adverse effects is the most critical step in determining the type studies required for approval. Since it is not expected that all the desired information will be readily available or may be from 'imperfect' studies, judgemental decisions will be required. Applicants are encouraged to check with the FDA, at this stage to arrive at an understanding as to what, if any, clinical studies may be required.

In developing a controlled release drug delivery system (defined as the dosage form and dosage regimen), it is important to look at the input function, i.e., cumulative amount of drug in the body at any given time if allowed to enter the body, but not leave. While this is not a regulatory requirement, it is instructive since it permits focusing on the absorption process without having to worry about the complexities and variabilities of the elimination process.

Most oral controlled release formulations have input functions that are combinations of zero-order and first-order. First order absorption has the disadvantage that when the dosage interval is less than four times the half life of the drug, there **must** be a "gut residual" (2), i.e., an amount of drug still remaining in the gut at the time the next dose is given. Given the complexities of gut motility, gastric retention, etc., it is very likely that this will contribute to the variability of the drug blood levels generated, or even decreased drug bioavailability (Fig. 2 and 3). Performing an analyses, (e.g., a Wagner Nelson or Loo Riegelman calculation) to determine the "fraction of the amount absorbed" versus time hours, enables the determination of the gut residual remaining to be absorbed during the next dosing interval(s). The larger the gut residual, the greater will be the potential for day to day variation of blood levels.

Other potential problems of oral controlled release dosage forms include gastrointestinal transit time, decreased bioavailability because of site specific absorption, decreased bioavailability due to increased first pass metabolism, dose dumping, food effects and diurnal variation.

Although it has been reported that GI transit in a given population varies from 5 to 35 hours, recent data indicates that intestinal transit time in any given individual, in a given set of conditions, does not vary much. On the

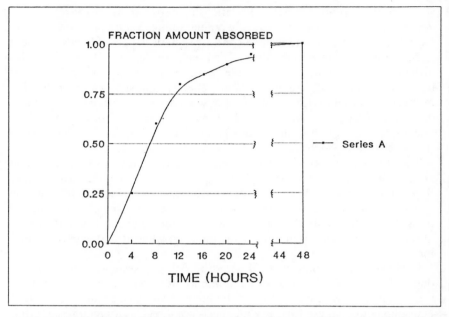

Fig. 2: Fraction of the amount absorbed plot of drug associated with acceptable C_{min} steady state variation. Fraction of the amount absorbed plot calculated by the Wagner-Nelson Method. Note that, in this simulation based on real data, only 95% of the drug dosed is absorbed within the 24 hour dosage interval. The additional 5% will be absorbed within the next dosage interval.

other hand, factors influencing gastric emptying may severely affect gastric transit. Food administration which delays the 'housekeeper wave' causing a significant delay in gastric emptying is a major influence. A high fat meal delays gastric emptying for 3–5 hours. The extent and significance of these influences may be substantial and are largely at this point in time, unknown. The data indicate it may be both dosage form and drug specific.

4. Decreased systemic availability due to incomplete absorption or increased first pass metabolism

Many controlled release products are somewhat less bioavailable than their immediate release counterparts. This can be due to incomplete release from the dosage form or release at such a slow rate that the drug has passed the optimal sites of absorption.

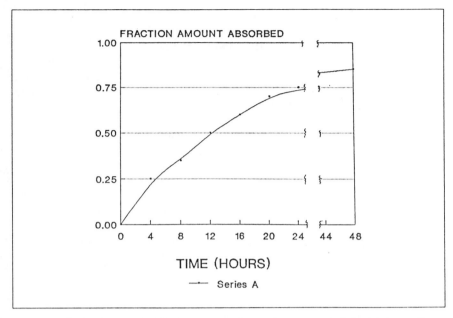

Fig. 3: Fraction of the amount absorbed plot of drug associated with large C_min steady state variation. Fraction of the amount absorbed plot calculated by the Wagner-Nelson Method. Note that, in this simulation based on real data, only 75% of drug dosed is absorbed within the 24 hour dosage interval. The additional 25% will be absorbed in the next two dosage intervals.

The fraction of drug metabolized during first pass by hepatic or intestinal enzymes can be altered by dosage forms which markedly alter the rate at which the drug is presented to the enzyme system(s). If the enzyme systems are saturable, then a slower rate of presentation may result in a greater fraction of drug metabolized. Phenytoin is an example (3). The steady-state plasma levels of phenytoin observed with equal doses of the prolonged release product are less than for the prompt release product. The difference in plasma levels appears not to be due to decreased absorption, but rather increased metabolism as the amount of total drug in the urine is the same for both formulations. Because of its narrow therapeutic ratio, nonlinear kinetics and different clinical uses, the USP recognizes two dosage forms: prompt (for immediate release) and extended (for controlled release) (4).

5. Effects of diurnal variation

There are examples in which the pattern of release of controlled release products varies, depending upon the time that the product was administered (morning versus evening). The reasons for these diurnal differences are not clear. In some cases they may be simply related to the fact that the evening doses were given with meals. In other cases, however, the effect of meals can be ruled out and changes in G.I. motility or drug disposition at night may be the factor producing differences. Because of the potential for differences in AUC at different times of the day, it is necessary to sample the entire dosage period when testing a 24 hour product. Also if the product is to be given at night, it is necessary to test the product at night.

Osman, et al. (5), Sips, et al. (6), Leeds, et al. (7), Lagas and Jonkman (8), Pedersen (9) & Moeller-Petersen (10), Hendeles and Weinberger (11) and others have demonstrated that food may significantly increase, decrease or have no effect on drug release when administered with food versus administration under fasting conditions. In the case of theophylline, this appears to be dosage form specific.

6. Regulatory assessment of controlled release products

In order to gain FDA approval of New Drug Applications for a new chemical entity initially marketed in Controlled Release Dosage Forms (as with all other similar products) clinical studies in patients establishing the safety and efficacy of each particular dosage form are required. In addition, as a result of the FEDERAL REGISTER publication of January 7, 1977 on Drug Bioavailability, it is required that the bioavailability of each new dosage form be determined. The pharmacokinetic description of the absorption, distribution, metabolism and elimination of that particular chemical entity in that dosage form, and justification of the dosage regimen recommended in the labeling needs to be submitted.

As with new drugs in conventional dosage forms, data need to be submitted for regulatory approval of a controlled release drug product (or drug delivery system) to substantiate the clinical safety and efficacy (if not otherwise known), of the controlled release product and demonstration of its controlled drug release characteristics.

6.1 Demonstration of safety and efficacy of controlled release drugs

6.1.1 For drugs which have been approved by the FDA as safe and effective in conventional dosage forms, the Food and Drug Administration has taken the position that controlled clinical studies may be required to demonstrate the safety and efficacy of the drugs (already approved for use in conventional forms), in the controlled release formulation. For drugs like theophylline where the pharmacokinetic and pharmacodynamic relationship is well defined, they have accepted pharmacokinetic data in lieu of clinical trials. In any case, bioavailability data for the drug(s) in the controlled release formulation are required.

6.1.2 For drugs which have been previously approved as safe and effective in controlled release dosage forms, data are required to establish bioavailability comparability to an approved controlled release drug product. In this case, the labeling must be identical to the reference standard with regard to effectiveness and side effects. Without appropriate clinical studies to justify the change, the labeling cannot be modified to make any different claims in clinical effectiveness or side effects.

6.1.3 Single dose bioavailability studies are acceptable for determining the fraction of the amount absorbed, lack of dose dumping, lack of food effects, etc. Pharmacokinetic studies, performed under steady-state conditions are acceptable to demonstrate comparability to an approved immediate release drug product, occupancy time within a therapeutic window, percent fluctuation, etc., and are acceptable for supporting dosage administration labeling.

6.1.4 The optimum single dose study would be a three way crossover comparing a rapidly available dosage form (I.V. solution, oral solution, or a well characterized conventional dosage form), and the controlled release dosage form under fasting conditions with the controlled release dosage form administered immediately after the ingestion of a high fat meal.

The optimum multiple dose steady state design depends on whether data exist to establish that the conventional drug follows linear pharmacokinetics. When existing data establish that the immediate release product follows linear pharmacokinetics, a steady state study with the controlled release product at one dosage rate (preferably at the high end of usual dose rate range), using an immediate release formulation as the control, should at a minimum be conducted. Plasma concentrations over at least one dosage interval of the controlled release product should be measured in each leg of the crossover, although it may be preferable to measure concentrations over the entire day in each leg. The controlled release product would be acceptable if it produced the same equivalent AUC (using accepted FDA criteria) as the immediate release product and the degree of fluctuation for the modified release was comparable to or less than that for the immediate release product. The appropriate measurements would include, of course, unchanged drug and/or major active metabolites.

Where steady state comparison of the immediate release product at different dose rates is not available or where nonlinearity is exhibited, steady state crossover studies comparing the controlled release product with the immediate release product at two different dose rates should be conducted (one at the low end of the recommended dosing range and a second at the high end of the dosing range). For each of the comparisons the controlled release product must meet the same criteria in regard to AUC and fluctuation as specified above. If there are significant differences between the controlled release product and the immediate release product at either the high end or the low end of a dosing rate, this data alone would not serve as a basis of drug product approval.

With drugs having a narrow therapeutic index, it might be necessary to carry out more extensive plasma concentration measurements in patients to determine the potential for unusual drug release patterns. In these studies more than one measurement would be made to assess patient variability with both the controlled release and immediate release dosage forms.

6.2 Submitted data should provide assurance that:

6.2.1 A pharmacokinetic profile, including fraction of the amount absorbed (Wagner, Nelson, Loo Riegelman, etc.).

6.2.2 The drug product meets the controlled release claims made for it. If zero-order absorption is claimed, then an appropriately calculated input function should be provided to substantiate that the majority of the input function is zero-order.

6.2.3 The bioavailability profile established for the drug product rules out the occurrence of dose dumping (especially when dosed with a fatty meal).

6.2.4 Bioavailability data – either demonstrating comparability to the reference dosage form(s) with the same labeling, indications, and side effects; or lack of comparability to the reference dosage form. In the latter case data demonstrating safety and efficacy as well as different labeling will be required.

6.2.5 Where a therapeutic window exists, determination of percent of time the blood level remains in the therapeutic range, i.e., the "Therapeutic Occupancy Time."

6.2.6 Percent of fluctuation $\dfrac{C_{max} - C_{min}}{\dfrac{C_{max} + C_{min}}{2}}$

6.2.7 The drug product's steady-state performance is equivalent to a currently marketed conventional release, or a specified controlled release drug product containing the same active drug ingredient or therapeutic moiety, which is subject to an approved new drug application. Daily dosage must be comparable.

6.2.8 The drug product's formulation provides consistent pharmacokinetic performance between individual dosage units.

6.3 Recommended reference standard for comparative studies:

6.3.1 Either an intravenous solution or an oral solution or suspension of the same active drug ingredient or therapeutic moiety. If a suspension is used care must be taken that the suspension itself has adequate bioavailability.

6.3.2 A currently marketed, approved, conventional release drug product with defined biovailability and reproducibility, containing the same active drug ingredient or therapeutic moiety, or

6.3.3 A specified currently marketed controlled release drug product with defined reproducible bioavailability, subject to an approved new drug application containing the same active drug ingredient or therapeutic moiety.

6.3.4 In some instances (A) or (B) and (C) above may be required.

6.3.5 In order to avoid selection of an inappropriate reference, the Director, Division of Biopharmaceutics (or in the case of generic drugs, Director, Division of Bioequivalence), should be consulted before initiating studies.

Bioavailability data consisting of blood levels and/or urinary excretion rate profiles performed under steady-state conditions may be acceptable in lieu of clinical trials, if it can be demonstrated that the blood levels and/or urinary excretion rates are comparable to multiple doses of the same drug in appropriate conventional dosage forms, or to an equivalent dose of the same drug in appropriate controlled release dosage forms. In these cases, the labeling must clearly indicate that the recommended dosing regimen and the claims of effectiveness and side effects are identical with the reference dosage form. Because of the difficulty that may be encountered in frequent urine collection and the validity of urine data, urinary excretion rate profiles, as a condition for bioavailability comparability should be cleared with the Division Director before protocol approval.

Any labeling claims of clinical advantage, such as greater effectiveness and/or reduced incidence of side effects, must be substantiated by appropriate well-controlled clinical studies. Clinical testing may be required unless there is substantial evidence that the drug's effectiveness is related to the absolute blood level achieved at steady-state, rather than the rate of change of drug level.

The controlled release formulation developed should aim to accomplish two important objectives: (1) It should allow a maximum possible percentage of the dose in the formulation to be absorbed; and (2) it should be capable of minimizing patient-to-patient variability.

6.4 Specific types of in vivo studies

6.4.1 Fasted single dose studies

a. For a controlled release dosage form the major concern is the fraction of drug absorbed and the rate of release (i. e., the input function).
b. The Wagner-Nelson or Loo-Riegelman equation needs to be applied to single dose study data, so as to obtain the fraction of the amount absorbed per unit time where appropriate.

6.4.2 Post prandial study:

The conditions of the post prandial study should be the same as for the fasted study except for drug dosing. In this instance, the controlled release product should be administered immediately after the ingestion of a standard breakfast. We recommend 2 medium sized eggs, 2 strips bacon, toast with butter, 2 to 4 or. hash brown potatoes and a glass of whole milk. Subjects should then fast for 4 hour.

6.4.3 Multiple dose steady-state studies

It is not really possible for a controlled release drug product to be properly evaluated by single dose administration alone. For prescription products there is a need to determine whether the controlled release dosage can achieve well-defined therapeutic plasma levels or that the plasma levels obtained are comparable to those generated by an immediate release dosage form administered to healthy volunteers or patients as labelled.

It should be emphasized that bioequivalence employing exact superimposition of plasma levels need not be demonstrated for purposes of product approval; for by definition, the rate of absorption for a controlled release dosage form will differ appreciably relative to immediate release dosage forms, and may differ from other controlled release dosage forms. What needs to be established, is satisfactory bioavailability and pharmacokinetics to support drug labeling. The following criteria should be met:

a. Satisfactory steady-state plasma levels should be obtained with the test drug and reference drug in sufficient patients or volunteers to warrant a comparability determination.
b. Determination of steady-state should be established by comparison of 'C_{min}' (trough values) on three or more consecutive days. Fluctuation greater than 15% should be closely examined for food effect, diurnal variation, achievement of steady-state, etc.
c. Failure to achieve satisfactory steady-state in a large percentage of subjects tested may indicate possible lack of patient compliance, failure of dosage form performance, etc.
d. Comparison of pharmacokinetic parameters, e. g., 'C_{min}', 'AUC' values, etc., should be limited only to subjects who achieve steady-state conditions.

e. Comparison of 'AUC' during a dosing interval is only proper if both the test drug and reference drug are at steady-state.

f. Where it exists, consideration must be given to the "therapeutic window." One is concerned in steady-state, as to what percentage of time the drug concentration lies within the "therapeutic window." The "occupancy time." The occupancy time for each subject and for mean data should be determined.

6.5 Demonstration of a products controlled release nature

It is necessary (where possible) to demonstrate the controlled release nature of a drug from a controlled release formulation by both **in vitro** and **in vivo** methods. Formulators of controlled release drug products are urged to develop reproducible and sensitive **in vitro** methods to characterize the release mechanisms of the controlled release drug products. The **in vitro** test developed should be utilized to access the bioavailability of the controlled release dosage form by "red flagging" possible lot-to-lot **in vivo** performance differences.

6.6 Biopharmaceutic considerations

While it is generally accepted that the present state of technology does not permit meaningful in vitro versus in vivo correlations for extended release dosage forms, adequately validated in vitro dissolution testing can be developed to facilitate process control to enable the determination of some of the final product specifications. The Controlled Release Workshop recommended that "to determine the suitability of this in vitro test, the relationship of the results obtained with this test to the actual in vivo absorption characteristics of the test products should be established in a small group of human subjects."

It recommended that the in vitro test was desirable for the purposes of (a) providing necessary process control and stability determinations of the relevant release characteristics, and (b) facilitating certain regulatory determinations and judgments, concerning minor formulations changes, site of manufacturing changes, etc. It recommended: (a) Preparation of at least three dosage formulations with different biopharmaceutic characteristics (changes in in vitro dissolution of these test dosage forms being accomplished by changing only these process and component variables that are likely to be varied under normal manufacturing conditions); (b) Development of an appropriate in vitro test capable of distinguishing between these formulations; and (c) Determination of the absorption characteristics of these formulations in a small group of human subjects. The in vitro drug release kinetics of the dosage form intended to be marketed should be characterized as a function of medium pH, rate of agitation, and possibly also medium composition (e.g., surfactants and bile salts). Since the knowledge of controlled release product in vitro/in vivo correlation development and test is still evolving, alternative approaches to this problem should be explored and should be considered by the Agency on their merits.

The key elements for dissolution are:
a) Reproducibility of the method.
b) Proper choice of media.
c) Maintenance of sink conditions.
d) Control of solution hydrodynamics.
e) Dissolution rate as a function of pH ranging from pH 1 to pH 8, including several intermediate values, preferably as topographic dissolution characterization (12, 13, 14).
f) Selection of the most discriminating variables (media, pH, rotation speed, etc.) as the basis for the dissolution test and specifications.

The dissolution procedure should establish:
a) Lack of dose dumping – indicated by a narrow limit on the one hour dissolution specification.
b) Controlled release characteristics – by employing additional sampling windows over time. (Narrow limits with an appropriate Q value system will control the degree of first order release).
c) Complete drug release – indicated by a 75–80% minimum release specification at the last sampling interval.
d) Dosage form pH dependence/independence indicated by percent dissolution in water, appropriate buffer, gastric,* and simulated intestinal* fluid.
* Minus enzymes

6.7 Consideration for specialized controlled release drug delivery systems

In recent years, novel drug delivery systems have evolved which are designed to deliver drugs at pre-defined rates over a prolonged period of time. Included among these are Ocusert[R], Oros[R], copper and progesterone releasing IUDs, and transdermal systems. All such new drug delivery systems are considered new drugs requiring full new drug applications (NDA) as a basis of drug approval.

In addition to safety and efficacy considerations, which includes an understanding of the drug input function, plasma blood level oscillation, and the drugs pharmacodynamics, there are biopharmaceutic and pharmacokinetic issues that need to be addressed by the manufacturer such as:
a) Reproducibility of the new drug delivery system by **in vivo** or **in vitro** studies.
b) A defined bioavailability profile which rules out dose dumping.
c) Demonstration of reasonably good absorption relative to an appropriate

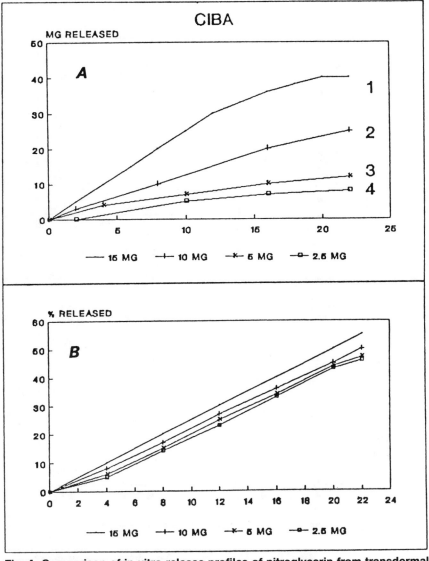

Fig. 4: Comparison of in-vitro release profiles of nitroglycerin from transdermal patches, given as
· milligrams per patch (A, C, and E)
· % label claim release (B, D, and F)

Figure 4a: CIBA'S PATCHES

Curve 1, 15   mg (30 cm²)   Curve 3, 5   mg (10 cm²)
Curve 2, 10   mg (20 cm²)   Curve 4, 2.5 mg (5 cm²)

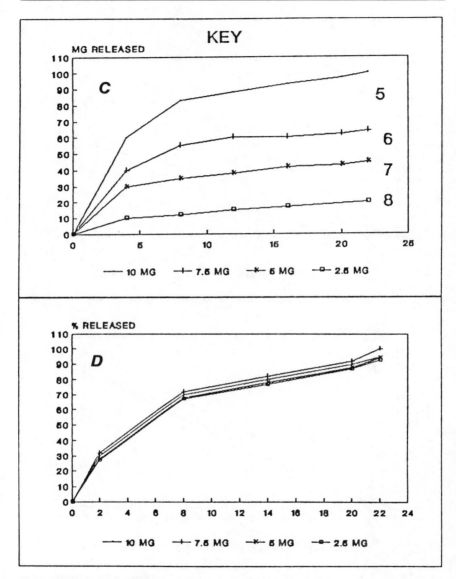

Figure 4b: KEY'S PATCHES
Curve 5, 10   mg (20 cm²)
Curve 6,   7.5 mg (15 cm²)
Curve 7,   5   mg (10 cm²)
Curve 8,   2.5 mg (5 cm²)

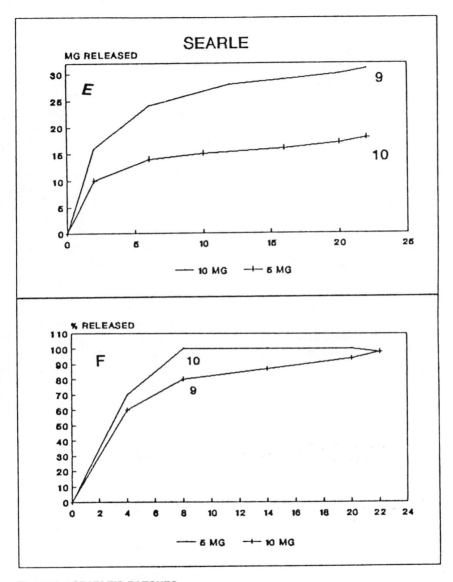

Figure 4c: SEARLE'S PATCHES
Curve 9, 10   mg (16 cm²)
Curve 10, 5   mg (8 cm²)

standard and which considers important elements, e.g., obviating of first pass gut or liver metabolism.

d) A well-defined pharmacokinetic profile to support drug labeling.

e) **In vitro** characterization (where possible).

The toxicologic and clinical requirements for systemically effective dermal-transdermal drugs should parallel other systemic drugs of the same pharmacological class. From a biopharmaceutic point of view, there is a need to define the bioavailability/pharmacokinetics relative to an intravenous dose, ideally, or an oral dose if an I. V. dose is not feasible. As well as defining the pharmacokinetic profile of a new drug delivery system, it is necessary to demonstrate the reproducibility of such systems. This involves both demonstrating the reproducibility of the dosage form as well as drug delivery to the patient. The latter can be achieved by comparison of the blood level profiles of different batches of a new drug delivery system in the same patients or by **in vitro** dissolution testing be used to define reproducibility. FDA's Division of Biopharmaceutics has studied this and developed satisfactory dissolution procedures for nitroglycerine transdermal patches (Fig. 4). The data show consistent dissolution performance among product lines and even establish dose proportional dissolution within the same product line (15).

In summary, the justification for regulatory approval of controlled release formulations of established and new drug entities should be based solely on the scientific documentation for that drug in terms of safety and efficacy. Regulatory approval of a controlled release drug product in terms of bioavailability needs demonstration of the controlled release nature of the product and in many cases bay be used in lieu of clinical studies.

References

(1) Controlled Release Dosage Forms "Issues and Controversies". (Sept. 29–Oct. 1, 1985) Cosponsored by Food and Drug Administration, Academy of Pharmaceutical Science, and American Association for Clinical Pharmacology & Therapeutics, Washington, DC

(2) Barr, W. H.: Bioavailability of Solid Oral Dosage Forms and Clinical Response to Drug Therapy in **Current Consepts in the Pharmaceutical Sciences; Dosage Form Design and Bioavailability;** Ed. James Swarbrick; Lea & Febiges; Phila., Pa.; 1973

(3) Gummitt, J., and Sawchuk, R. J.: FDA contract number 223–76–3019

(4) United States Pharmacopeial Convention publication; 1985 – USP XXI; published by USP, Rockville, Md

(5) Osman, M. A., Patel, R. B., Irwin, D. S., Welling, P. G.: Absorption of Theophylline from Enteric Coated and Sustained Release Formulations in Fasted and Non-Fasted Subjects: Biopharmaceutics and Drug Disposition 4, 63–72 (1983)

(6) Sips, A. P., Edelbroek, R. M., Kulstad, S., de Wolff, F. A., Dijkman, J. H.: Food Does Not Affect in Bioavailability of Theophylline from Theolin Retard. Eur. J. Clin. Pharmacol. 26, 405–407 (1984).

(7.) Leeds, N. H., Gal, P., Purohit, A. A., Walter, J. B.: Effect of Food on the Bioavailability and Pattern of Release of a Sustained Release Theophylline Tablet J. Clin. Pharmacol. 22, 196–200 (1982)

(8) Lagas, M., Jonkman, J. H. G.: Greatly Enhanced Bioavailability of Theophylline on Postprandial Administration of a Sustained Release Tablet. Eur. J. Clin. Pharmacol. 24. 761–767 (1983)

(9) Pedersen, S., Moeller-Petersen, J.: Influence of Food on the Absorption Rate and Bioavailability of a Sustained Release Theophylline Preparation. Allergy 37, 531–534 (1982)

(10) Pedersen, S., and Moeller-Petersen, J.: Erratic Absorption of a Slow Release Theophylline Sprinkle Product. Pediatrics 74, 534–538 (1984)

(11) Hendeles, L., Weinberger, M., Milavetz, G., Hill, M., Vaughan, L.: Food Induced "Dose Dumping" from a Once-a-Day Theophylline Product as a Cause of Theophylline Toxicity. Chest 87, (6) 758–765 (1985)

(12) Skelly, J. P., Yamamoto, L. A., Shah, V. P., Yau, M. K. and Barr, W. H.: Topographical Dissolution Characterization for Controlled Release Products – A New Technique Drug Development and Industrial Pharmacy; Submitted

(13) Skelly, J. P., Yau, M. K., Elkins, J. S., Yamamoto, L. A., Shah, V. P., and Barr, W. H.: In Vitro Topographical Characterization as a Predictor of In Vivo Controlled Release Quinidine Gluconate Bioavailability; Drug Development and Industrial Pharmacy; Submitted

(14) Skelly, J. P.: Bioavailability of Sustained Release Dosage Forms – Relationship with In Vitro Dissolution; Academy of Pharmaceutical Sciences Meeting, Minneapolis, Minn.; 1985

(15) Shah, V. P., Tynes, N., Yamamoto, L. A., Skelly, J. P.: In Vitro Dissolution Profile of Transdermal Nitroglycerin Patches Using Paddle Method. International Journal of Pharmaceutics 32, 243 (1986)

XI. Regulatory Recommendations in Europe on Investigation and Evaluation of Oral Controlled Release Products

A. G. Rauws, M. Olling, Bilthoven

Summary

To ensure safety and efficacy of controlled release products it is primarily necessary to require pharmacokinetic proof or their bioavailability and controlled release characteristics. Besides, eventual special claims related to the controlled release character may have to be substantiated by pharmacokinetic or clinical studies. Within Europe only in the Nordic countries, in the United Kingdom and in the German Democratic Republic recommendations on requirements on investigation and evaluation of controlled release-products are in force that are based on bioavailability studies. The working party "Efficacy" of the CPMP is preparing an controlled release-recommendation. The same is done by the Committee for Evaluation of Medicines in the Netherlands. The Nordic and UK-Recommendations are discussed, as are some considerations on requirements for controlled release-products and on measures of controlled release character, needed to discriminate between controlled release-products and just slowly released conventional products.

1. General considerations

The development of controlled release (CR) preparations started in the early fifties. Its primary aim was to decrease dosing frequency (1, 2). In a later phase, when plasma concentrations of medicines became a measure of pharmacotherapeutic quality, the aim shifted to the attainment of safe, effective and constant plasma concentrations especially in chronic therapy. "The flatter, the better!" New materials and technologies were introduced to improve the properties of controlled release preparations (e. g. the durette matrix) and in the last years innovative forms were developed, partly with complicated structures and built-in energy sources (e. g. oral osmotic systems). The aim of these special designs is to approach as much as possible a zero order release process (Fig. 1). One may now consider controlled release preparations as a subgroup of the therapeutic systems, the oral group.

So one may define oral controlled release preparations by using Heilmann's definition for therapeutic systems (3) in a slightly modified form: "An oral controlled release preparation is a pharmaceutical dosage form that after oral administration releases a medicine continuously in a predetermined pattern for a fixed period of time".

The aims in development of controlled release preparations are the following:
1. Constancy of plasma concentrations within the therapeutic range.
2. Implicit: Prevention of side effects.
3. Decrease of dosing frequency.
4. Implicit: Better patient compliance.

The implicit aims 2 and 4 have sneaked into the thinking, about controlled release-products, without having been thoroughly tested as feasible. Meanwhile it appears that the attainment of these aims is difficult to demonstrate. They are much influenced by patient variables. But as claims they will have to be proven.

2. Regulatory considerations

Newly developed controlled release preparations generally contain active substances, whose properties are well documented. The dosage form however brings with it the allegation of special claims. In this aspect there is a large difference between conventional products and controlled release preparations. The bioavailability of a conventional form is proven by a straightfor-

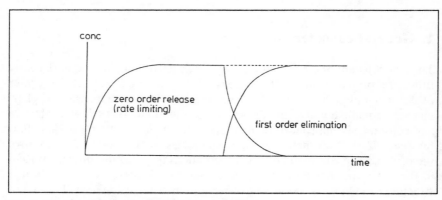

Fig. 1: Idealized controlled-release preparation.

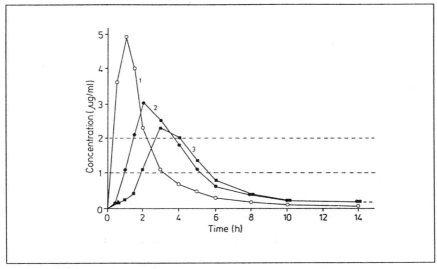

Fig. 2: Plasma concentration time course after conventional (1) and slow release indomethacine preparations (2 and 3) (From Bechgaard et al., ref. 14).

ward biopharmaceutical quality test "in vivo". The claims connected with the controlled release formulation however surpass the usual biopharmaceutical test system. In the application for registration of controlled release products these claims will therefore have to be substantiated by separate pharmaceutical, pharmacokinetic and also pharmacotherapeutic studies. This is not just overregulation. The experience with organic nitrate controlled release products has shown that pharmacokinetic data were not enough (4). The once a day theophylline preparations were inferior to the twice a day analogues until one matched their plasma level fluctuation with the circadian rhythm in sensitivity to bronchoconstriction (5).

At the present many products are on the market, whose controlled release properties are only marginal (Fig. 2). They release their active substance just more slowly than their conventional analogues (Fig. 3) as may be seen if they are shifted in a way to have their t_{max}-values coincide. They do not differ from them otherways, than by a lower maximal plasma concentration and a later time of attainment of that maximum. It is important to develop criteria which allow a clear discrimination between real controlled release products (Fig. 4) and essentially slow conventional products (Fig. 2). Furtheron notes for guidance on controlled release preparations should set standards for investigation of the product and for evaluation of the claims made. All regulation should be viewed as a consequence of the fundamental requirements of **safety** and **efficacy.**

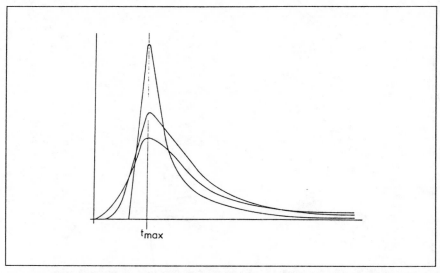

Fig. 3: Curves of Figure 2 shown with coinciding t_{max}, to illustrate similarity of elimination half-lives.

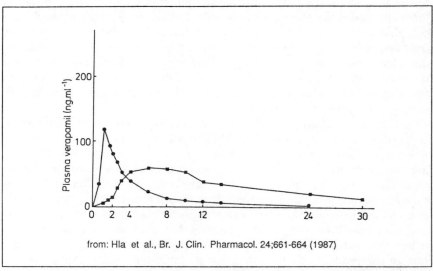

from: Hla et al., Br. J. Clin. Pharmacol. 24;661-664 (1987)

Fig. 4: Plasma concentration time course after conventional (●) and controlled-release (■) verapanil preparations. (From Hla et al., ref. 15).